THE XXL SYNDROME

Obesity, diabetes, heart attacks: potassium can change everything

It's natural, it's my health

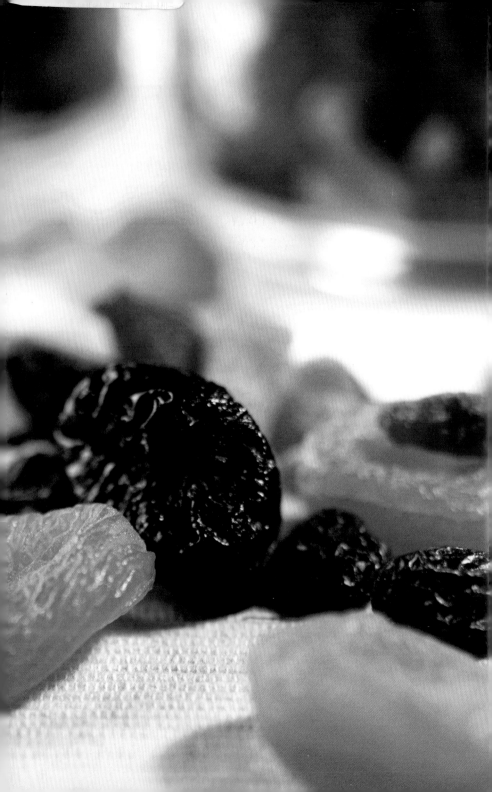

THE XXL SYNDROME

**Top up your Energy
Don't let your engine idle.
Take Potassium,
the Mineral that revs up
your cells**

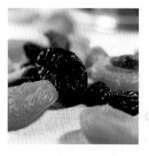

Dr Max Rombi

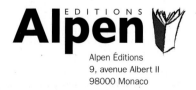

EDITIONS
Alpen

Alpen Éditions
9, avenue Albert II
98000 Monaco

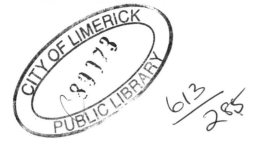

613/285

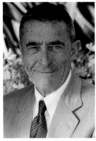

In 1956, Dr MAX ROMBI qualified as a Veterinary Surgeon in Toulouse. After studying biochemistry and pharmacology, he worked on Research & Development in the pharmaceutical industry. He then became an entrepreneur, creating the Virbac Veterinary Company in 1967. Finally, in 1980, he set up Laboratoires Arkopharma, which have since become world leaders in phytotherapy and alternative medicine. Arkocaps have enjoyed a success that has spread worldwide. Dr Rombi believes that people must always be informed so that they can take their own health in hand. This is why he has written this book, following so many others, to explain the usefulness of potassium (that rejected mineral) and the dangers of salt.

This book is going to revolutionise medicine.

Exclusive copyrights:

©Alpen Éditions
9, avenue Albert II
98000 Monaco
Tel: +377 97 77 62 10
Fax: +377 97 77 62 11
web: www.alpen.mc

Printed in Italy
ISBN: 978-2-35934-042-6

A Word from the Author

*We had thought of calling this book **Potassium, the Forgotten Mineral**.*

*Then we thought of calling it **Potassium, the Rejected Mineral**.*

For example, it is never mentioned in the RDA (Recommended Daily Allowance) lists. You will find calcium there, and magnesium, zinc, selenium, sodium chloride, but never potassium, as if it were unimportant and unnecessary.

Yes, potassium really is a rejected mineral.

Now potassium is the mineral most abundantly present in the body (about 140 g).
More so than calcium or phosphorus, which make up the bones, more so than sodium, that is present in the blood and the lymph.

Potassium is the mineral that is most important to the body. It governs the mineral balance in the cells. Without it, there would be no life, and we shall see that it is the way it competes with sodium, that dominant mineral used in excessive amounts in our modern world, that is at the root of a syndrome that causes many illnesses. There are so many of these illnesses, and they cover such a wide field, that we have decided to call this the XXL syndrome, which is the title finally given to this book.

Never forget, potassium must never be forgotten.

NOTE:

The information contained in this book cannot replace an authoritative opinion. Before embarking on any self-medication, consult a doctor or a qualified pharmacist.

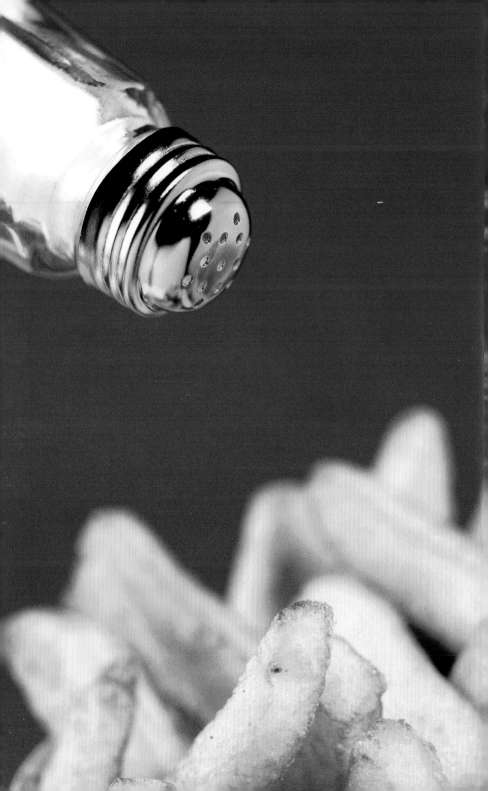

Introduction

How can anyone fail to be concerned at the worldwide increase in illnesses such as diabetes, hypertension, excess weight and obesity, cardiovascular disease, hypercholesterolemia, and asthma as well?
How can anyone fail to be surprised at the rise in nervous and mental illnesses: not feeling well, nervous fatigue, nervous depression, not to mention Alzheimer's disease.

All these epidemics (because they really are epidemics, even if not all these ills are infectious) have to be caused by something, several things. Dietary errors? Unsuitable lifestyle? No doubt.
We are eating more, and eating more and more foods with a high fat content. We are taking less and less exercise, we go everywhere by car, we take the lift rather than walk upstairs. But what is the deep-lying cause of these epidemics?

It was by studying the research carried out by Jens C. Skou (Nobel Prize for Chemistry 1997), Peter Agre and Roderick MacKinnon (Nobel Prize for Chemistry 2003), who worked on the channels enabling our cells to live, subsequently discovering that our cells have a very different mineral composition from our blood (our cells contain 28 times more potassium than the blood and 15 times less sodium than the blood),

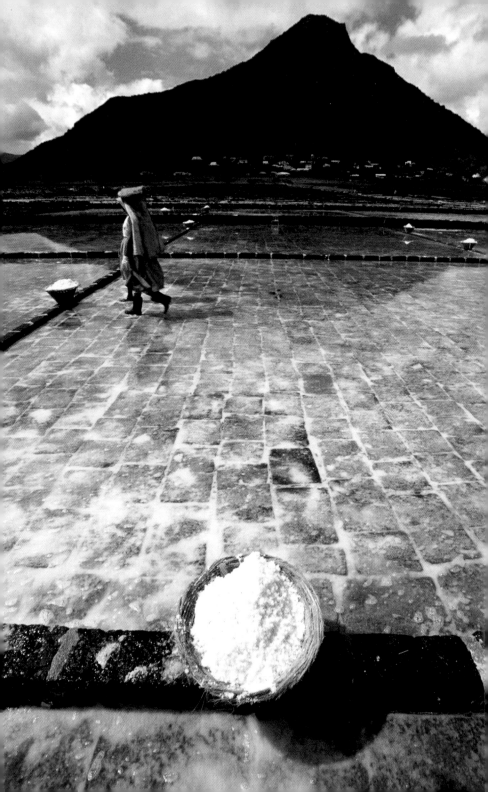

and finally by noting that a mineral balance
had been upset (salt* intake is colossal in all forms
of human society whereas potassium, sodium's first
cousin, is completely forgotten) that we realised
how these epidemics have spread
and are spreading throughout the world.

This book is thus the result of a police investigation
into what is to blame for these epidemics
and the biological reactions that cause these illnesses,
which all have a common factor:
too much salt, not enough potassium.

Let's start our investigation…

* We need to know that table salt is sodium chloride, chemical formula NaCl;
salt contains 60% chlorine (Cl) and 40% sodium (Na, from the Latin *natrium*).

CONTENTS

THE XXL SYNDROME

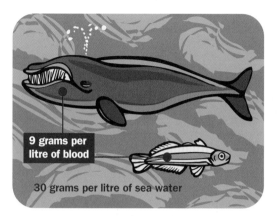

9 grams per litre of blood

30 grams per litre of sea water

The Fight for Life

We readily talk about life being a battle. When they say that, some people think of the battle to find food, others of the battle against infection... whereas in reality, there is a ceaseless battle that not many people have thought about: the battle to regulate the mineral composition of our cells.

Fish are not salty either

Poach a cod fillet and it will seem tasteless because it is not salty. It is this peculiarity possessed by fish that Dr Bombard took advantage of when, in 1952, he crossed the Atlantic without provisions or water, living solely off the juices from the fish he caught. Thus, like mammals, fish eliminate the salt that they swallow and keep their blood salt level at 9 g per litre. Their cells, like ours, contain a lot of potassium and little sodium.

The prowess of animals that live in sea water

All marine animals have the same peculiarity: the mineral composition of their internal medium is very different from that of the sea water that surrounds them. Their blood contains 9 g of salt per litre, although these animals live in sea water that contains 30 to 38 g per litre, i.e. three times as much! Whales, seals, dolphins, killer whales and, of course, fish, constantly swallow sea water and consequently a lot of salt. Under these conditions, they are faced with a considerable difficulty: keeping at the same blood composition despite the continuous influx of salt into their internal medium. For these animals, it is a ceaseless battle, the fight for life.

Our cells
are like a fish in sea water

Like all animals, our blood contains 9 g of salt per litre. Fortunately, we don't drink sea water but for our cells, immersed in our blood, our internal sea, the battle is the same. They, too, have to fight constantly because the mineral composition of their internal medium is totally different from that of the blood that surrounds them. The intracellular medium is much less salty. There is 15 times less sodium in our cells than in the blood and 11 times less chlorine. On the other hand, there is 28 times more potassium. According to some scientists, the mineral composition of our cells is close to that of a primitive sea at the time when the first living cells were formed. It has not changed since, whereas the sea has become considerably more salty. But never mind, however this difference came about, the battle is on: our cells, with their low salt, high potassium contents, have to fight continually to eject the sodium and chlorine which ceaselessly enter them.

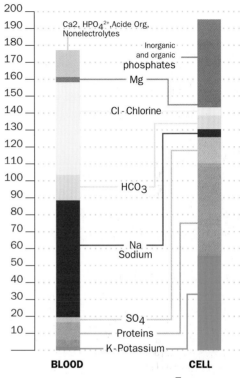

Comparison of the composition of the blood and the intracellular fluid (in mEq/l)

Ca2, HPO$_4^{2+}$,Acide Org, Nonelectrolytes
Inorganic and organic phosphates
Mg
Cl - Chlorine
HCO$_3$
Na Sodium
SO$_4$
Proteins
K - Potassium

BLOOD   CELL

11 times more chlorine in the blood than in the cell

15 times more sodium in the blood than in the cell

28 times more potassium in the cell than in the blood

The whole purpose of this book is to show that if the fight goes against our cells, if they do not manage to eliminate the excess sodium, it is a catastrophe. The cells become unwell. They lose their vitality. The vital processes are hindered and serious illnesses ensue.

Castaways: their Tragedy

Man cannot live by drinking sea water. Castaways who drink sea water die after 2 or 3 days. This sums up the tragedy suffered by castaways, floating on a vast stretch of water that they cannot drink.

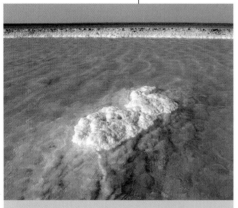

Sodium: the Sea's Mineral

Even though there is a great abundance of sodium on land, it is above all the sea's mineral. It is found in the form of a salt, sodium chloride. On land, it is present in a few minerals such as feldspaths, which are sodium silicates. It is also found in the large salt deposits that are worked in mines worldwide (deposits that were once seas and are now dry). The chemical symbol for sodium is Na (from the Latin *natrium*).

Dr McCance, Professor of Experimental Medicine at Cambridge (England) has carried out research on castaways. During the Second World War, he was Chairman of the British Admiralty Sub-committee responsible for saving the lives of the hundreds of castaways drifting in lifeboats or on rafts after their ships had been sunk by German submarines. He studied volunteers in lifeboats in temperate, arctic and tropical seas and came to the firm conclusion that sea water could not be used to supplement a limited supply of drinking water. Reports from survivors showed that those who had drunk sea water became delirious sooner and could more readily topple over and disappear overboard. Sea water contains such a high salt concentration that our kidneys cannot tolerate it; this is why, when it is drunk, it has the effect of removing all water from the body, making dehydration worse[1].

Chemically, what is salt?

Chemists call it sodium chloride, chemical formula NaCl, consisting of a sodium atom: Na and a chlorine atom: Cl.

In solution in water, the salt molecule cleaves and releases two atoms: Na on the one hand, Cl on the other. When separation occurs, the sodium atom loses an electron (and thus becomes positively charged: Na^+) whereas the chlorine atom gains an electron and becomes negatively charged: Cl^-.

These electrically charged atoms are known as ions and they behave differently according to how they are charged. When a direct current is passed through a salt solution, for example, the negative ions (Cl^-) go to the positively charged anode: these ions will then be termed **anions**. Whereas the positive ions (Na^+) go to the cathode; these are the **cations**.

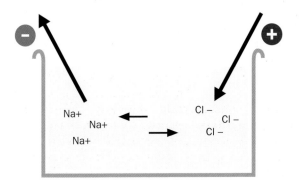

Potassium: the earth mineral

Potassium has a high presence in all emerged continents. This is an element that is essential to life. It is very important to plant growth, whereas salt is inimical to plants – only a few plants, called halophilic, can grow in salty soils. Potassium is also found in potash, deposits of which are mined to manufacture fertilisers. The word potash is derived from "pot" and "ash", the ash left in a pot after burning plants. All plants contain a lot of potassium. The chemical symbol for potassium is K (in Latin, *kalium*).

I'm sodium, you're potassium

Potassium and sodium are the Laurel and Hardy of our health. We cannot do without either of them, both have a part to play. One does not go without the other and each has its place in the body. This is the price of our health.

Sodium outside the cell

Sodium comes from the salt that we add to our food. It is the principal cation (*see p.15*) in the **extracellular** medium, i.e. the blood and lymph. It regulates the body's water content; when sodium is lost, water is lost; when sodium is absorbed, water is retained. It is due to sodium that our blood volume is constant, as well as the blood pH, i.e. its acid or basic nature. Finally, sodium acts as a co-transporter, i.e. it enables nutrients to penetrate into the cells. Like a sort of "taxi", sodium, through the channels, takes glucose, amino acids and many other nutrients that the cell needs in order to live, with it through the membrane.

Potassium within

We are provided with potassium by fruit, vegetables and all animal meats and fish. It is the principal cation (*see p.15*) in the **intracellular** medium. It performs the same functions inside the cell as sodium does outside it; it regulates the cell's water content and its pH. Potassium activates many enzymes inside the cell to enable proteins to be produced from amino acids and glucose to be converted into glycogen, the stored sugar for the muscles and the liver.

Water in the body

Water accounts for about 60% of bodyweight. It is divided between the intracellular fluid (the water contained in the cells) and the extracellular fluid in which the cells are immersed, i.e. the blood and lymph. Two-thirds of body water is inside the cells, the remaining one-third outside. There is thus nearly **twice as much potassium as sodium** in the body.

Sodium and potassium are crucially important to excitable cells

The term excitable cells is applied to **neurons** that transmit the nervous impulse, **muscle cells** such as those of the myocardium that cause the heart to beat and **glandular cells** such as those of the pancreas that secrete insulin. These cells have a common feature, they are able to develop a bioelectrical signal and this signal essentially depends on the potassium-sodium exchanges between the inside and the outside of the cell. It is due to movement of these ions on either side of the cell membrane (through specific channels) that the nerve cells communicate and the muscles contract.

Mineral composition, in grams per litre

	Blood	Inside the cells
Sodium	3.40	0.230
Potassium	0.195	5.50
Magnesium	0.078	0.012
Calcium	0.078	traces
Chlorine	3.9	0.350

► 28 times more potassium in the cell than in the blood
► 15 times more sodium in the blood than in the cell
► 11 times more chlorine in the blood than in the cell

Potassium in the body

The body of a normal man weighing 70 kg contains about 140 g of potassium. Ninety per cent of the potassium is inside the cells (9% in the connective tissue and the bones, 1% in the plasma). It is above all present in the muscle cells (40% of total potassium), the liver cells and the red blood cells. Essentially, we obtain it from fruit and vegetables but also from the flesh of the animals that we eat – meat or fish – since living cells contain an abundance of potassium. Potassium is largely eliminated in the urine (80-90%) and a little in the stools as well.

Sodium in the body

The body of a normal man weighing 70 kg contains about 93 g of sodium, including 45 g in the bones, 38 g in the extracellular fluid and 10 g in the intracellular fluid. It comes from the salt that we add to our food. Normally, the amount of sodium eliminated in the urine is equal to the amount ingested. If a person adds no salt to his food, almost no sodium is found in the urine because the kidneys retain it. Genetically, we are programmed to save sodium and re-absorb it through the kidneys. This is why adding a lot of salt to food increases our body sodium.

Too much Sodium, not enough Potassium

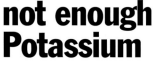

Sodium and potassium are two minerals that are very important to our bodies. They have an essential part to play and we need them to be supplied in strictly accurate proportions. To function properly, we need a little sodium and a lot of potassium.

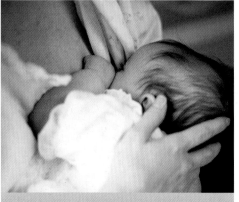

A low-sodium, high-potassium ancestral diet

Vegetables contain only traces of sodium, whereas their potassium content is high (20 mg of sodium and 1000-5000 mg of potassium per kg).

Animal products (meat or fish) account for the intracellular medium, low in sodium and high in potassium (100-500 mg of sodium and 1000-4000 mg of potassium per kg).

Mother's milk, the basic food during the early months of life, contains little sodium and appreciable quantities of potassium (300-400 mg of sodium, 1000-2000 mg of potassium per kg).

Return to the roots

For thousands of years, we ate foods that were low in sodium and high in potassium. Bearing in mind that our most direct ancestor, Cro-Magnon Man, appeared some 30,000 to 50,000 years ago, our species has, for more than **90% of its history**, adopted a diet based on game, fish, fruit, vegetables, nuts and seeds containing 5 to 10 times more potassium than sodium. In the beginning, therefore, man was getting **little salt**, 2 g of sodium per day, and a **lot of potassium**, about 12 g per day. Salt made its apparition in the diet when man became sedentarised. As he discovered salt's virtues for preserving food, he also discovered that it gave food a good flavour. Since then, the dietary sodium/potassium ratio has gradually been reversed.

Recent decades have seen the advent of ready-meals (with salt carefully added by the agrifood industry) and, simultaneously, a vertical fall in the consumption of fresh produce. Now, modern man eats 10 g of salt a day, sometimes much more, and he takes in no more than 2 g of potassium a day. Nowadays, therefore, we take in **2 to 4 times more sodium than potassium**.

Difficult to adjust

On the evolutionary scale, therefore, our diet has changed abruptly, but what about us? Well, not all that much. Our bodies function in exactly the same way as those of our remote ancestors. Moreover, as the prehistoric diet contained little salt, we are genetically programmed to reabsorb sodium: 95% of it is recovered by the kidneys when supplies are limited. Conversely, the body has not provided any potassium-saving system. Once ingested, potassium is absorbed then filtered by the kidneys and eliminated in the urine.

From a physiological point of view, this imbalance between sodium and potassium is bound to have repercussions. These two minerals are intimately linked and if we do not get supplies in the proper proportions, sooner or later illnesses are liable to appear. But let us pursue our investigation…

When we eat fresh, raw, unprocessed foods, it is impossible to take in more sodium than potassium.

The *paradoxical mineral*

It may seem surprising that potassium, which is the most important mineral in our cells, is so disregarded and used so little in our diet. Nobody says anything about it, nobody knows anything about it, and yet it is the most important element in our mineral life and our life, period. It is astonishing to note that no-one has ever emphasized the high potassium content in our cells or the need for an input of this mineral to keep them balanced. More seriously, potassium is a demonised mineral. The medical profession and pharmacists regard it as a dangerous mineral that must be handled with great care. For example, potassium injected by the intravenous route is said to be highly toxic. This example is tendentious, since even mineral water, injected intravenously, can be highly toxic by causing red blood cells to burst. Conversely, it may be felt surprising that such large quantities of sodium are ingested (salt is added to all our food) when, eaten in such proportions, it is the source of so many health problems. A great many people regard sodium as a friend and potassium as an enemy. What are the reasons behind this disinformation?

Sodium's real danger to our cells

Our cells need sodium to function. But when there is an excess of sodium, it causes very serious disorders.

We are made up of billions of cells and it is the existence of all these cells that accounts for our body's life. These cells have a life of their own. They are surrounded by a membrane that defines their internal medium and isolates them from the external medium, blood and lymph. It is in the blood and lymph that all the nutrients necessary to the cells circulate: oxygen, glucose, amino acids (constituents of proteins), minerals such as phosphorus, magnesium, vitamins and, of course, potassium.

How do these nutrients get through the membrane?

The membranes of our cells contain channels through which nutrients can pass.
Nevertheless, for all these molecules to be able to get in, they have to have recourse to a "taxi" that facilitates their entry; more often than not, this is sodium. Thus every time a nutrient penetrates into a cell, two sodium atoms go with it and enter at the same time.

However, while most of the nutrients consumed by the cell are converted by it (glucose is converted into carbon dioxide, amino acids produce proteins), when we take in too much salt, the sodium atoms accumulate and after a while, the cell contains too many of them.

Glucose and sodium transport in the epithelial cells of the intestine

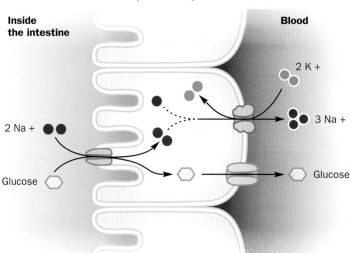

The sodium concentration increases, consequently the cell attracts water and swells (see the detailed explanation of osmotic pressure in the ensuing pages). As it already contains a lot of sodium, it is difficult for it to take in any more. It stops taking in further nutrients, despite the fact that it needs them. It thus finds itself living in slow motion, as if it were asphyxiated. Then it stops functioning. Sometimes it may even stop living!

A multiplicity of consequences

When our cells reach this state of living in slow motion, it has repercussions on the whole of our body. For example: if cells contain too much sodium and no longer assimilate any glucose, the latter will accumulate in the blood, leading to diabetes. Another example: if the cells in our arteries swell because of a surplus of sodium, compression of all these swollen cells will lead to an increase in blood pressure. There will be hypertension.

These are only two examples among so many others. There are numerous scenarios showing that the unbelievable dysfunctional states that medicine calls fatigue, diabetes, asthma, hypertension, etc., are in fact simply a direct consequence of an excess of sodium in our cells and excessive swelling of many of them.

Metabolic blockage under the magnifying glass:
why does excess sodium make cells swell?

To understand this properly, let's do a bit of chemistry revision...

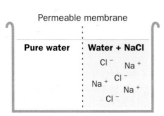

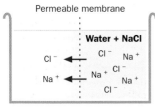

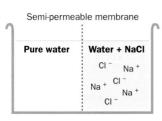

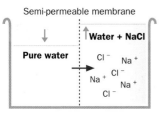

Take two compartments separated by a membrane: one contains pure water, the other a saline solution. The salt molecule ($NaCl$) in the water disintegrates, producing two ions: Na^+ and Cl^-. If the membrane is permeable (lets the ions and the water pass), the system evolves until the ion concentrations are equal on either side of the membrane. When equilibrium is reached, the water concentration is also identical on both sides.

If the membrane is semi-permeable (it allows water to pass but not ions), the system tends to evolve towards the same state of equilibrium of concentrations. But as the ions are no longer getting through the membrane, only the water passes through: this water diffusion is known as **osmosis**.

Diffusion is possible only from areas where there is a high concentration of diffusible molecule (in our case water) to areas where there is a low concentration of that molecule. The water will thus go from the compartment where it is pure to the compartment where its concentration is lower (because the ions are there and they attract water by a magnetic force which we call osmotic pressure). This water flow is reflected by an increase in the volume of solution in the compartment containing the ions.

To resist this change in volume, pressure would have to be applied to the compartment containing the saline solution so as to cancel out the water flow. This pressure corresponds to the **osmotic pressure**

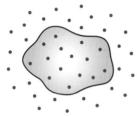

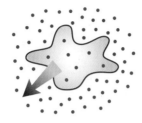

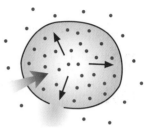

a) Osmotic equilibrium:
salt concentration identical
inside the red blood cell
and outside

b) More salt outside:
water is attracted to the outside
of the red blood cell,
which contracts.

c) Less salt outside:
water is attracted to the inside
of the red blood cell,
which swells and may burst.

of the solution. It thus measures the "water pulling power" from a concentrated solution..

What happens in our cells?

Our cell membranes behave like semi-permeable membranes and allow only water to pass. The intra-cellular medium contains numerous ions in solution in the water, including sodium and chlorine. When red blood cells are placed in pure, thus salt-free, water, they attract water because the water in their internal medium contains more salt. The red blood cells swell and may even burst (c). Conversely, if red blood cells are placed in sea water (a concentrated saline solution containing 30 grams per litre), the red blood cell loses its water, which this time is attracted by the sea water. It then contracts and becomes smaller (b). Then if red blood cells are placed in an isotonic solution (9 g NaCl per litre), the red cell remains a normal size (a).

Never any pure water by infusion

After a surgical operation or a haemorrhage, in short whenever there is severe loss of blood, blood volume has to be restored quickly. Pure water, free from mineral salts, cannot be injected into the blood because the red blood cells would burst. This is why physiological saline solution, i.e. water containing 9 grams of salt per litre, is injected.

The consequence of excess salt in our food

We have seen that when we take in too much salt, the intracellular medium accumulates sodium and with it larger molecules such as glucose and amino acids. This creates an imbalance on either side of the membrane. The water concentration becomes lower inside the cells than outside. Water will therefore penetrate into the cells by osmosis. The cells swell and we shall see that this change in volume has direct effects on their vital activities.

Metabolic blockage under the magnifying glass:
why do swollen cells live in slow motion?

There is a direct link between the volume of a cell and its activity.

When the cells swell, the energy vanishes.

The cell is the site of intense activity. Like a little self-contained factory, it manufactures molecules and at the same time supplies the energy necessary for this purpose. The synthetic reactions (anabolism) need energy in order to take place: using simple molecules, which can be regarded as bricks, the cell builds larger molecules. It is the degradation reactions (catabolism) that supply the necessary energy: the cell "breaks" molecules into smaller elements, which liberates energy. Anabolism and catabolism make up what is called metabolism.

In a healthy cell, the synthetic reactions are always coupled to degradation reactions. But as soon as the cell swells, this equilibrium between synthesis and degradation is broken. An increase in volume is perceived by the cell as a message asking it to synthesize more. The energy demand becomes greater than the supply, with the result that the cell's energy reserves dwindle. Sooner or later, the cell's metabolism will be blocked.

Explanations

Metabolism influences the cell's volume, and vice versa

• Experimentally, when a cell's metabolism is inhibited, an accumulation of sodium in the cell follows, which has the effect of attracting molecules of water (by osmosis) and, unfailingly, the cell swells. This has been demonstrated with brain, kidney, liver and muscle cells [2].

• The reverse is true. Any change in cell volume has a direct influence on its metabolism. This mechanism has been widely studied on liver cells. Nowadays we know that when liver cells are swollen, glycogen synthesis from glucose is stimulated, as is protein synthesis from amino acids (anabolism). Conversely, the glycogen and

Anabolism and Catabolism

The life of our cells is ceaselessly in equilibrium between anabolism, a biosynthetic process, and catabolism, a degradation process. Anabolism is characterised by the synthesis of molecules in the cell, the production of reserve bodies. If you break a leg, your broken bone will, for several weeks, be the site of frantic anabolism in order to ossify the bone and repair the fracture. Similarly, when you put on weight and your cells store fats, you are in a state of anabolism. Conversely, degrading reserve molecules in order to obtain small molecules for burning to obtain energy is catabolism. Losing weight, for example, is a typical catabolic process. Therefore, never forget this: when our cells swell because of excess salt within those cells, all catabolism is blocked. The cells go into anabolism and store up reserves. Overall, this means that the cells become even larger, they store fats and have no energy. Result: great fatigue and weight gain.

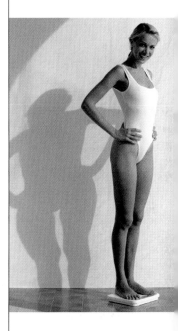

protein degradation reactions are inhibited (catabolism). This means that in a swollen cell, anabolism takes precedence over catabolism: the cell stores, makes reserves, but no longer has the energy needed to burn up these reserves. Under these conditions, the cell's energy gradually decreases: the cell lives in slow motion [3].

To sum up, when a cell increases in volume, its metabolism is slowed. This is true of liver cells but also of all our cells.

Exchanging sodium for potassium: the Na/K pump

To combat an accumulation of sodium that is harmful to cells, nature has organised matters well. She has endowed them with a pump: the sodium-potassium pump (also abbreviated to Na/K pump). But if it is to be efficient, this pump needs to have enough potassium available to it.

They are everywhere

Na/K pumps are omnipresent in the cells of different animal species. They are even found in the most rudimentary living things such as bacteria, entities consisting of a single cell. In man, according to the organ involved, there may be between 800,000 and 30 million pumps per cell. In the kidneys or the intestinal mucosa, the pumps are literally caked together and indeed they are an energy-engulfing pit since they burn up nearly 25% of the cell's energy reserves and up to 70% in the nerve cells.

Some fifty years ago, researchers demonstrated the existence of a set of biochemical processes in the cell membrane making it possible to extract sodium ions from the cell and put in potassium ions.

In all our cells, there are membrane proteins which work similarly to a pump. These pumps are responsible for removing sodium from the cells and replacing it with potassium: three sodium ions come out against two potassium ions that go in.

A vital pump

The cell, by expelling sodium, sees its volume reduced. Moreover, by expelling more sodium than they take in potassium, the pumps create a potential difference between the outside and the inside of the cell and behave like mini-generators, batteries of a kind, supplying the cell with energy. Thus, up to 70% of a cell's energy may come from these pumps. This is the case, for example, with neurons and the cells in the glands that

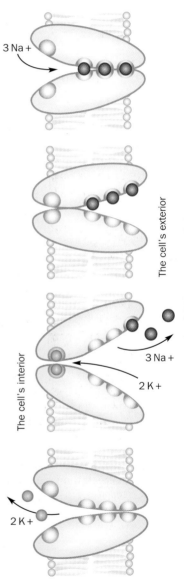

The sodium-potassium pump
The inside of the cell is very low in sodium;
on the other hand, it is very high in potassium.
This difference is the result of active
ion transport through the cell membrane
due to the sodium-potassium pump.
It is a membrane protein which,
following various contortions,
expels three sodium ions outside the cell
and brings two potassium ions inside the cell.
When this cycle, which takes barely
a few milliseconds, is complete,
the pump is ready for a further cycle.

3 Na +

The cell's exterior

The cell's interior

3 Na +

2 K +

2 K +

secrete our hormones. These pumps are essential to life. They enable our cells to feed. If these pumps stop working, it is certain death. But for them to function properly, the cells have to have enough potassium available to them in the blood, and this is normally supplied by our food. To eliminate sodium from our cells, we have a crucial need for potassium in our food and in our blood.

The most important battle in our life

If you are accustomed not to take much salt in your food and if you spontaneously eat plenty of fruit and vegetables, thus plenty of potassium, every-thing will be fine. But if you take in too much salt and not much potassium, as is the case nowadays for most of us, the battle is lost, unless we have inherited especially efficient genes (very effective Na/K pump). The Na/K pumps will not be able to do their work properly. Sodium will accumulate in the cell, leading to the metabolic blockage that we have described in previous pages.

The XXL Syndrome

In 1988, an American specialist at Stanford University, Dr. Gerald Reaven, described the X syndrome for the first time. There is nothing exotic or even exceptional about this syndrome, he said, since it affects 60 to 75 million Americans. In reality, insulin resistance is concealed behind this term, which sounds as if it comes straight out of science fiction.

The X syndrome is diagnosed when a person presents with at least two of the following signs: abdominal obesity, high triglyceride level, too-low level of HDL-cholesterol (the "good cholesterol"), hypertension, high insulin level when fasting. People affected by the X syndrome are at greater risk of developing Type II diabetes and cardiovascular disease. They also have a higher probability of dying prematurely of these diseases.

But while cardiovascular disease and diabetes are indeed developed-country diseases, the list is far from exhaustive. It leaves out cancers (breast, prostate, colon cancer), obesity, osteoporosis, Alzheimer's disease, nervous depression, asthma, fatigue, etc., all of which suggests that the heart of the problem goes far beyond resistance to insulin.

This poor health situation is caused by **blockage of the metabolism** in all our cells. We believe it is the breakdown of the Na/K pump in each of the body's cells which, because of an excess of sodium and a deficiency of potassium, can no longer ensure

Illnesses caused by the XXL Syndrome

Cardiovascular diseases: hypertension, strokes, cardiac insufficiency, cardiovascular problems in postmenopausal women.

Metabolic illnesses: Type 2 diabetes, excess weight, obesity, hypercholesterolemia.

Nervous disorders: nervous depression, bipolar syndrome, Alzheimer's disease, epilepsy.

Respiratory illnesses: asthma, chronic obstructive bronchopneumopathy.

Digestive diseases: stomach cancer, ulcers, irritable bowel syndrome.

Fatigue

Osteoporosis

assimilation of glucose and other nutrients. The cells are swollen, they live in slow motion and no longer perform their functions properly.

As all illnesses caused by this metabolic blockage are far more numerous than those mentioned in the case of the X syndrome, we decided to call this metabolic blockage **the XXL syndrome**.

A concatenation of consequences...

The slowing of metabolism in each of our cells is reflected by a lack of energy in the whole body. You feel very tired. The XXL syndrome is also reflected by weight gain, with fats being stored, and circulatory problems added to the cardiovascular risk from the X syndrome, leading to the heart being overworked. Hypertrophy of the cardiac muscle then precedes cardiac insufficiency...

In short, a whole series of developed-country illnesses whose incidence increases ceaselessly despite medical progress and the medicines available to us.

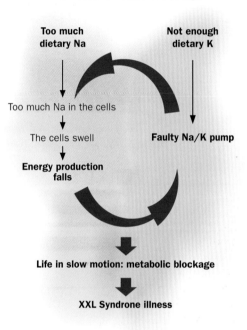

Salt/potassium imbalance: a vicious circle that leads to metabolic blockage

Too much dietary Na

Not enough dietary K

Too much Na in the cells

The cells swell

Faulty Na/K pump

Energy production falls

Life in slow motion: metabolic blockage

XXL Syndrone illness

The XXL syndrome is characterised by metabolic blockage in all our cells, as a result of excess sodium in them and a lack of potassium to expel the sodium. This is not an illness like influenza which is caused by a virus that comes into conflict with our immune system and disappears in a week or two. It is a set of changes in each of our cells that triggers and promotes the XXL syndrome illnesses.

THE XXL SYNDROME ILLNESSES

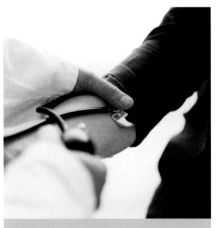

Hypertension, a silent disorder

You don't "suffer" from hypertension. Its effects are stealthy, latent. Common in developed countries, it affects 15-20% of the population and especially the over-65s.

What is hypertension?

Blood pressure is the force exerted by the blood on the walls of the arteries. Blood pressure is expressed by two figures, e.g. 140/90 or "140 over 90" because the pressure exerted on the arteries by the blood varies. The highest pressure is reached when the heart contracts. Between contractions, when the heart is at rest, the pressure falls to its lowest level. Doctors call the highest figure "systolic pressure" and the lowest figure "diastolic pressure". Normal blood pressure in adults is below 120/80 mm Hg. High blood pressure is 140/90 mm Hg or higher.

The cells of the arteries are in direct contact with high-sodium blood. In a person affected by the XXL syndrome, the Na/K pump cannot fulfil its function properly. Sodium accumulates inside the cells. The latter engorge with water and become turgescent. By swelling in this way, they compress the blood. In the muscle cells of the vessels, this is reflected by a fall in their reactivity. The arteries harden. They are less supple and offer more resistance to the blood flow, which causes blood pressure to rise.

When the Na/K pump is jammed

In order to gain a good understanding of the XXL syndrome, it is useful to see what happens when the Na/K pump is prevented chemically from working. Some medicines used in cardiology, such as digoxin or ouabain, are able to bind to these pumps, thus preventing them from working. In the vessels, the "blockage" is reflected by a constriction (vasoconstriction) and this is exactly what happens with the XXL syndrome..

Pressure increases with age.
True, but not everywhere…

The figures for normal pressure depend on the patient's age. The rule for making the calculation is as follows: the person's age + 100. For example, a young man of 20 should have 120 mm of mercury for systolic pressure. In practice, this value is expressed in cm of mercury. Normal pressure for a 20-year-old is therefore 12. It will be 13 for a 30-year-old, 14 for a 40-year-old, and so on. It is therefore regarded as normal for pressure to increase with age. However, this is only true of populations which have access to salt. In societies which consume no salt, this correlation is not found.

Why is high blood pressure harmful?

When blood pressure reaches a level that is too high, and stays there, it may, in the long run, lead to lesions of the arteries and the sensitive internal organs such as the heart, brain, kidneys or some parts of the eye. Hypertension also forces the heart to work harder, which may damage it in the long term. Finally, it is harmful because it roughens the lining of the arteries, which is usually smooth as a mirror. Fats and cholesterol are then able more easily to embed themselves into the artery walls and end up blocking the arteries. Being hypertensive thus increases the risk of having a heart attack, a stroke and renal failure.

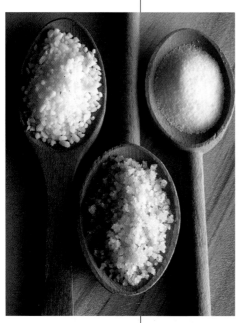

Guilty of causing Hypertension: salt

As long as 3700 years ago, Chinese doctors noted that "when large amounts of salt are absorbed, the pulse becomes stronger and harder".

It was not until 1904 that two French doctors, Ambard and Beaujard, again saw the connection between salt intake and hypertension. But their research convinced nobody. In 1922, two English doctors, Allen and Shenil, carried out clinical trials on 180 people with severe hypertension and showed that excess salt intake heightens blood pressure. Nevertheless, despite all this evidence, the world medical community was not convinced. Recently, more and more studies have been performed and there is no longer any room for doubt.

The INTERSALT Study

The most complete epidemiological study so far is incontestably the INTERSALT study which compared more than 10,000 people from 32 different countries, divided into 52 samples. This study clearly shows that the more salt is taken in, the more blood pressure increases with age. But in that case what happens when intake is reduced? Well, pressure decreases. In 1960, the

Japanese were eating 18 g of salt per day; in 1989, this had fallen to 14 g. Result: the adult blood pressure figures fell, as did deaths from strokes. The blood pressure reduction was even more spectacular in children. In 1968, a big information campaign on the dangers of excessive salt intake, aimed at middle-aged people, was launched in Belgium. A reduction from 16 to 11 g per day for men and 12 to 9 g for women produced a drop in blood pressure figures both in people under medical treatment and untreated.

With potassium, it's even better!

If the potassium supply to hypertensives is increased, blood pressure falls even more.

More than 33 studies have been conducted using potassium supplements on people suffering from hypertension. Collectively, these studies indicate that potassium causes a significant reduction in blood pressure. The decrease is greater in people who take large amounts of salt.

The reason for this is simple: when potassium activates the Na/K pump, the arteries, arterioles and capillaries dilate, which has direct repercussions on blood pressure.

Potassium, as effective as medication

A team of English nutritionists (King's College, London) gave 30 people, free from apparent health problems, 1 g/day of a potassium supplement (equivalent to the amount of potassium contained in five portions of fresh fruit and vegetables). After six weeks of supplementation, the blood pressure of these people had fallen significantly compared with the placebo group:

- 7.60 mm of mercury for systolic pressure,

- 6.46 mm of mercury for diastolic pressure.

The researchers concluded that "potassium lowers blood pressure efficiently, as efficiently as antihypertensive medication"[4].

The Ultimate Proof: DASH

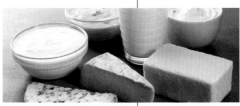

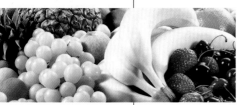

The DASH (*Dietary Approaches to Stop Hypertension*) study was launched to ascertain whether a diet can avoid the need for medication. It succeeded beyond all hopes.

DASH studied the effects on blood pressure of several dietary combinations. Three types of diet were offered to 459 adults with normal to moderately high blood pressure.

• A control group followed a reference diet: 4 portions of fruit or vegetables, half a portion of dairy produce per day.

• A second group was offered 8.5 portions of fruit and vegetables, thus containing more potassium and magnesium, the remainder being the same.

• A third group, called the "combination" group, followed a diet with a very high fruit and vegetable content (10 portions), with reduced-fat dairy produce, less saturated fat and less cholesterol.

Salt intake was the same for all three groups, about 3 g per day.

Diet as effective as medication

Compared with the group on the reference diet, the people in the "combination diet" group saw their blood pressure fall more significantly than those in the "fruit and vegetable" group.

Moreover, this diet proved to be as effective on hypertensives as expensive, sometimes dangerous, medication!

Everyone on a salt-free diet

In the context of the follow-up to the DASH study, the researchers asked 417 people to modulate their sodium intake.

One group took 3.5 g a day, another 2.3 g and the third 1.2 g. The lower the salt intake, the greater the fall in blood pressure, even when it was not initially raised. It decreased at all ages and regardless of the sex and skin colour of those taking part. "We can now say that a reduction in salt intake has beneficial effects on everyone, not only hypertensives" commented Professor Claude Lenfant, Director of the American National Heart, Lung and Blood Institute at Bethesda (Maryland, USA).

Hypertension in figures

USA

• About 65 million American adults now have high blood pressure – 30 percent more than the 50 million who did in the previous decade.

• One in five Americans (and one in four adults) has high blood pressure but because there are no symptoms, nearly one-third of these people don't know they have it.

• Of all people with high blood pressure, only 34 percent are on medication and have it controlled. 25 percent are on medication but don't have it under control, and 11 percent aren't on medication.

• From 1991 to 2001 the death rate from high blood pressure increased 36.4 percent, but the actual number of deaths rose 53.0 percent.

• High blood pressure killed 46,765 Americans in 2001.

Source: American Heart Association.
High blood pressure statistics
http://216.185.112.5/presenter.jhtml?identifier=4621

EUROPE

• Hypertension affects 50 million Europeans.

• Taking all age groups together, the incidence of hypertension is highest in Germany (55%), followed by Finland (49%), Spain (47%), the United Kingdom (42%), Sweden and Italy (38%).

• According to the Monica study, blood pressure levels are generally lower in South European countries than in those in North and East Europe.

Strokes
and Heart Attacks

A rise in blood pressure is the main risk factor in strokes and heart attacks, the two most important causes of death worldwide. Could the XXL syndrome be a link in the chain?

A stroke occurs when the blood flow encounters an obstacle (blood clot or broken blood vessel) which obstructs its passage towards the different parts of the brain. Deprived of oxygen, the nerve cells in the affected brain area cannot function and die in a few minutes. The damage is irreversible because the dead brain cells are not replaced. When the same problem occurs in the heart (constriction or clot formation in the coronary arteries), the result is a heart attack (infarction). The cardiac muscle is damaged, which may be fatal.

Potassium deficiency, look out, danger!

This is the conclusion reached by researchers from Queen's Medical Center in Honolulu who monitored 5600 people over the age of 65 for a period of years (4 to 8 years) in the United States. The researchers regularly measured the serum potassium level and the dietary potassium supply. When analysing the data collected, they noted that the lower the potassium level, which applies notably to people on diuretics, the higher the risk of a stroke. The tendency is the same for people who take in little potassium[5].

The XXL syndrome promotes blood clot formation

The blood circulates starting from the heart, then in the arteries. It further goes through a set of small arterioles that penetrate our tissues. Finally, these arterioles end in capillaries. These are very small channels that go through all our organs and supply blood to the smallest recesses of our bodies. These capillaries are very fine and have a **diameter of 2 to 4 thousandths of a millimetre**. Plasma enters the capillaries easily, but red blood cells have difficulty because, with a

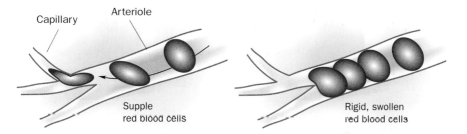

Capillary

Arteriole

Supple
red blood cells

Rigid, swollen
red blood cells

In order to enter the capillaries, red blood cells have to be very supple

diameter of 8 thousandths of a millimetre, they are larger than the capillaries. To get in, they have to twist and turn. Obviously they do it, because otherwise we could not exist. However, when there is excess salt and a deficit of potassium, its cellular exchange currency, the red blood cells, heavy with salt and swollen, get into the capillaries with difficulty or not at all. The effect of this is to create little clots that will stop blood from circulating. If this happens in the brain, it is a stroke; if it happens in the cardiac muscle, it is a heart attack.

The XXL syndrome reduces artery diameter

The artery cells are in direct contact with the high-sodium blood. In a person with the XXL syndrome, the Na/K pump does not completely fulfil its function. Sodium accumulates in the cells. They engorge with water and become turgescent. As they swell, the cells reduce the diameter of the arteries and check blood flow.

Too much salt promotes strokes

Although the Chinese had already noted the triple relationship between salt intake, pulse rigidity and strokes, formal proof was provided by epidemiological studies. The most conclusive is still the INTERSALT study, performed on a worldwide scale: the greater the salt intake, the higher the blood pressure and the greater the risk of a heart attack or stroke.

Pasteur had stroke problems twice. At the end of his life, his right arm was paralysed. President Roosevelt and Stalin, who had hypertension, both died of a cerebral embolism. The Yalta Agreements followed them even to the grave...

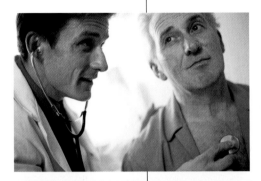

Cardiac insufficiency and left ventricular hypertrophy

Sodium-potassium exchanges play an important part in cardiac muscle contraction. Too much sodium, not enough potassium and the heart suffers.

Cardiac insufficiency in figures

USA

• Nearly 5 million Americans are living with heart failure, which is one of the most common reasons that people over age 65 are hospitalised, according to the American Heart Association.

• 50% of them die within 5 years of being diagnosed.

• 550,000 new cases are diagnosed each year.

• A person age 40 or older has a one-in-five chance of developing congestive heart failure.*

• The annual cost of treating heart failure is estimated at 40 billion dollars, It is the disease that costs the USA more than any other.

* Lloyd-Jones DM: *Lifetime risk for developing congestive heart failure.* Circulation 2002 ; 106 : 3068-3072.

Europe

• The number of people in Europe with heart failure is estimated at 14 million.

• The incidence of heart failure could increase by 70% by 2010.

• In the United Kingdom, 1.5 million people will be affected in 2015!

The heart is a muscle that pumps blood and circulates it through the lungs for it to take up oxygen and then throughout the body for it to provide the organs with the oxygen and nutrients needed for their metabolism. As with all muscle cells, heart cells contract due to movement of sodium and potassium ions on either side of the membrane. Discrete changes in the intracellular/extracellular potassium ratio may have a considerable influence on impulse generation and cardiac contraction. Under these conditions, the XXL syndrome has catastrophic consequences: slowing of the Na/K pump affects the quality of sodium-potassium exchanges. The heart does not contract properly (heart rate disorders). Its capacity for pumping blood to the tissues is reduced, it can no longer satisfy the body's requirements. This is cardiac insufficiency. To make up for this insufficiency, the heart hypertrophies in order to increase its working capacity. Initially, this hypertrophy is beneficial, since it makes it possible to face up to an abnormal situation, but in the end it becomes deleterious because it tends to aggravate the cardiac insufficiency. This is the vicious circle.

A heart as big as that

Epidemiological studies have shown that people who have a high-salt diet more often present with left ventricular hypertrophy, apart from any associated pathology. Some even conclude that ingesting salt is as decisive as hypertension in the development of left ventricular hypertrophy[6].
The red blood cells are bigger than normal. They circulate badly in the capillaries; the heart is therefore obliged to strain to circulate them and it hypertrophies.

Potassium for all!

Some scientists suggest that patients suffering from congestive heart failure (right and left ventricles) should systematically be given potassium supplementation even if their blood potassium level is normal.[7,8]

Potassium, magnesium, phosphorus: the winning trio

People with cardiac insufficiency are very often short of magnesium. Magnesium is the second cellular cation in importance. Like potassium, it is plentiful in all vegetables. Magnesium is necessary to the working of the Na/K pump: it allows it to be supplied with energy (ATP (adenosine triphosphate) fixation to the enzyme). A magnesium deficiency has a tendency to aggravate the XXL syndrome: the intracellular medium becomes increasingly loaded with sodium and even poorer in potassium. A large number of studies support the utility of magnesium supplements to reduce the advance of atherosclerosis, platelet aggregation or vascular spasm and hypertension. Combining magnesium with potassium for the preventive or curative treatment of all the illnesses caused by the XXL syndrome seems entirely justified. Moreover, as the Na/K channel gets its energy from ATP, it is important also to ensure a sufficient supply of phosphorus, a high-energy mineral.

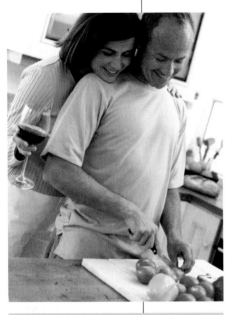

Potassium and *French paradox*

Despite risk factors identical to those of their European neighbours, French levels of cardio-vascular mortality are among the lowest on the planet. This French paradox, researchers believe, is largely explained by two dietary factors: omega-3 fatty acids and... **wine,** possibly indeed because of its potassium content (1 litre contains 800 mg!) In moderation (from one to three glasses per day), wine reduces the risk of heart attacks and strokes. When patients continue to drink wine after experiencing a heart attack, they run less risk of vascular complications.

It is easy to understand why peoples who grow vines, produce grapes and drink wine are in better vascular health than others. Is this not also the origin of the famous Cretan diet: wine + vegetables + sobriety?

Bad news for the arteries

Excess cholesterol is sensitive to oxidation by free radicals. Once oxidised, it accumulates in the artery walls and forms plaque that may block the arteries and lead to a heart attack. Could potassium play a part in this scenario?

Indispensable cholesterol

Cholesterol is a molecule classified as a fat but which has a different formula from fatty acids. It is a steroid. It has a twofold origin. The liver produces two-thirds of it, following a long chain of chemical reactions orchestrated by numerous enzymes, the chief of which is called HMG-CoA reductase. The remainder is supplied by foods of animal origin.

Cholesterol has several functions. The body uses it to make indispensable substances such as bile and sex hormones, among other things. But above all, it is one of the constituents of the membrane that covers all our cells. It has a structural rôle. It insinuates itself into the lipid bilayer, among the phospholipid molecules, and in a way constitutes the cell membrane's framework.

When the cells are swollen because of an excess of intracellular sodium and a shortage of potassium, the mechanical properties of the membranes change. The membranes are under pressure and therefore become rigid. The cholesterol no longer has enough room to insert itself among the phospholipids: it therefore returns into the blood stream, oxidises and promotes the formation of atheromatous plaques.

Potassium takes care of our arteries

Numerous studies in vitro and on animals suggest that high potassium intake gives protection against cardiovascular disease. Several studies[9] have shown that in hypertensive animals, potassium made it possible to reduce lipids in the blood and the vessels. Similarly, it prevents the macrophages from adhering to the artery wall. The macrophages are specialist cells responsible for clearing out LDL-cholesterol (the "bad" one). Unfortunately, when this cholesterol is oxidised, the macrophages discharge it into the arterial walls in the form of fats, and this contributes to forming atheromatous plaques. By preventing the macrophages from adhering to the walls, potassium could restrain cardiovascular diseases.

Other studies on animals have shown that potassium could reduce cholesterol deposits in the aorta.

Deep Vein Thrombosis

Potassium could be the great preventive remedy against DVT (Deep Vein Thrombosis), the thing Australians dread when they come to Europe and have to spend more than a day sitting in economy class in an aircraft.

Salt + sugar + fats: an explosive cocktail!

According to the INSEE (National Institute for Statistics and Economic Studies), the French are eating ever-decreasing amounts of fresh basic foodstuffs (consumption has fallen by 60%) and turning to ready-prepared meals (+ 5.5% per year since the 1960s) or highly processed products. In forty years, consumption of industrial confectionery and pastries has increased by 200%. Soft drink consumption has increased by 4.5% per year. Dairy produce, high in saturated fats, has made a spectacular leap: + 200%. This superabundance of highly processed, salted, sweetened and fatty foods, promotes the development of diseases related to dietary factors (our XXL syndrome) such as cardiovascular diseases, diabetes, cancer or obesity, which nowadays affects 10% of adults.

Menopause: the start of heart problems

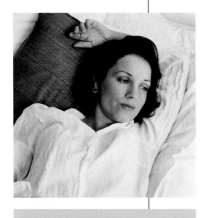

While cardiovascular diseases are unusual in women before the age of 50, the incidence curve for these diseases meets the men's about ten years after the menopause. Beyond 65, these diseases become the leading cause of female mortality.

Why this change?

Fifty, the age when the ovaries stop working and secretion of female hormones ceases. Women lose not only their fertility but also the protective effect that, until then, the estrogens exerted on the heart and vessels. These hormones have a beneficial effect on blood lipids and vascular tonicity. Take estradiol, the chief of these hormones. It has an antioxidant effect, i.e. it protects against free radicals; it also activates the potassium channels. It acts on the size of the cells and facilitates microcirculation by reducing the resistance to red blood cell circulation. Finally, it allows greater relaxation of the coronary arteries and the arterioles. [10, 11, 12, 13]

It is astonishing that these "secondary" activities by female hormones have never been brought to the forefront by the pharmaceutical companies that sell these hormones, no doubt because these activities devalue the hormone. On the other hand, to us, these "secondary" activities are of interest because we can replace

What changes at the menopause

As estrogen secretion decreases, women's levels of "bad" cholesterol (LDL-cholesterol) and triglycerides increase (+ 11%) while "good" cholesterol (HDL) decreases (- 10%). Blood pressure rises, too. The cardiovascular risk increases as weight rises and fat distribution changes (becoming preferentially located in the abdomen).

The solution: take antioxidants in the form of soya isoflavones (Phytosoya®) and eat a high-potassium diet.

them with products based on antioxidant plants that also activate the potassium channels, such as soya isoflavones and soya saponins.

Like an echo of the XXL syndrome

The XXL syndrome is not involved in the onset of the menopause but it does enable us to get a better insight into what happens deep within women's bodies at this time. Indeed, a fair number of the disorders they experience are related to those initiated by this syndrome. The lack of estrogens has the same kind of repercussions on the cells as an excess of sodium and a shortage of potassium.

For a long time, the only response from doctors has been to replace the missing hormones with synthetic hormones. This is the aim of the well-known HRT. Unfortunately, in recent years, many clinical trials conducted on very large cohorts have shown that these treatments are not without danger and that breast cancer and even (rather unexpectedly) cardiovascular complications could arise, with the result that gynaecologists no longer know what to do.

Tackling the menopause via the XXL syndrome is a highly interesting innovative approach since it opens the way to new treatments to help women to get through this change smoothly. Later on, we will take a detailed look at today's most significant alternatives to HRT (read pp. 92-93). These include potassium, of course, but also substances found in plants that are powerful Na/K pump activators (soya isoflavones).

Hot Flushes: a microcirculation problem

Hot flushes are explained by vaso-dilation (i.e. an increase in the calibre of the vessels in the skin) accompanied by a hot feeling all over the body and reddening of the face. Why does this vasodilation occur? In response to the fall in estrogens, the hypothalamus, a small region of the brain that controls body temperature, reacts as if the body were overheating: it orders the central nervous system to dissipate the supposedly excess heat by dilating the peripheral vessels and activating the sudorif-erous glands. For a short time now, a second mechanism has been suspected: the decrease in estro-gens could have a direct action on the skin arterioles, which would cause them to dilate. By activating the Na/K pump, potassium could limit this effect.

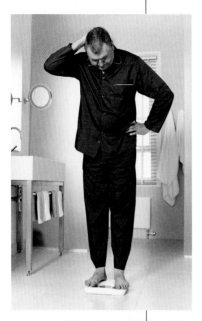

Obesity, a weighty problem

Obesity is gaining ground the whole time. Bad living habits, too-rich food, not enough exercise, faulty genes... all these probably come into the weight gain scenario, but none of these factors could cause such an epidemic on its own...

Salt promotes sugar absorption

One of the great dangers of salt is that it promotes sugar absorption. If there were no salt in the intestine, glucose would not be absorbed, or very little.

Sodium's first harmful effect: it stimulates glucose assimilation in the intestine. This was discovered a few years ago: glucose is absorbed by the epithelial cells in the intestine via a co-transporter which, when a glucose molecule is absorbed, passes in two sodium ions at the same time. This co-transporter is known as SGLT1. The glucose then goes into the blood by passive diffusion. Then it is converted into glycogen and stored in the liver and the muscles or converted into fat and stored in the fat cells (*see diagram on p.21*).

It can be seen immediately that the more sodium there is – it is known that salt is sodium chloride (NaCl) that in solution produces Cl^- and Na^+ in the intestine – the more sugar molecules bind to the sodium and consequently the more glucose is absorbed. Diabetics more than anyone must therefore be very careful about the amount of salt they ingest.

Similarly, the more carbohydrates we eat, the more glucose there is in the intestine and the more salt is absorbed. This vicious circle has dreadful effects on our health.

Salt stops cell metabolism, and they store more than they use

The second harmful effect that salt has, when it is combined with a shortage of potassium, is its general action on the size of our cells. Cells that contain too much sodium become turgescent and swell. Now, we have seen that according to numerous observations, an increase in cell volume increases anabolic activity (increases reserves and slows activity) (*read pp. 24-25*). When our cells are swollen and turgescent, due to an excess of sodium ions that increases osmotic pressure (and due to a lack of potassium to expel that sodium), they cease to work properly and they use every possible means to try to reduce their internal osmotic pressure to limit water penetration.

How do they manage this? By reducing the number of molecules dissolved in their intracellular fluid by manufacturing big, reserve molecules. For example: 50 glucose molecules together form a big glycogen molecule. Instead of 50 dissolved molecules, there is then only one. Similarly, 25 amino acids make a protein, which in terms of osmotic pressure counts as 1 instead of 25.

Thus by reducing the number of dissolved molecules in this way, our cells lower their osmotic pressure and swell less. The reverse of the medal is that the cell is then in storage mode and expends little energy. At whole-body level, this is reflected by weight gain and a patent lack of energy, an effect frequently felt by the obese, who are very often tired.

> If we want to lose weight, we have to burn up, produce energy and make the volume of our cells decrease by providing them with more potassium.

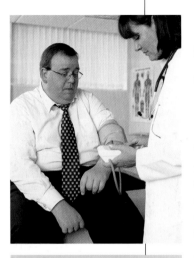

Obesity:
the XXL syndrome
in the dock

The XXL syndrome orchestrates weight gain like a maestro. It is involved in all levels of the process: first of all it stimulates fat storage, as we have just seen, then it slows energy expenditure. Under these conditions, resistance is difficult. Ineluctably, the scales tip in the wrong direction..

A fully-fledged illness

Obesity is an illness. Once it has set in, it develops of its own volition towards cardiac and vascular complications. It promotes resistance to insulin, which then leads to diabetes. In the joints, the weight of the unwanted kilos promotes arthrosis and pains in the joints.

The problem equated

Every day, 70% of our expenditure is due to basal metabolism. This expenditure is what we consume when we are doing nothing. It is the expenditure that is essential to ensure the working of our heart, our kidneys, our breathing, our brain and the life of all the cells in our body. 15% of energy expenditure comes from physical activity (every movement uses energy) and the last 15% is due to thermogenesis: we need energy to produce heat and maintain our body temperature at a constant level.

The XXL syndrome slows energy expenditure

The many studies carried out on the ion channels have provided a better understanding of how our cells work and a better apprehension of their energy balance. This is how researchers were able

15 %
thermogenesis

15 %
physical activity

70 %
basal
metabolism

to determine that the Na/K pump is at the root of 20 to 50% of the basal metabolism of our cells. Now, we have seen that it is essentially basal metabolism that governs energy expenditure (70% of energy expenditure). By reducing the working of this pump, the XXL syndrome decreases this expenditure directly. As the energy balance goes into deficit, the kilos pile on.

The obese are suffering from the XXL syndrome

Researchers have noted that in the obese, red blood cell Na/K pump activity was lower by 22% on average compared with people whose weight was normal. Researchers have also found an above-normal concentration of sodium inside these cells.[14]

> To lose weight, it is therefore necessary to revive all these cells and get calorie consumption going again. By taking potassium, Na/K pump activity is increased, sodium is expelled from the cells. The pump works better, nutrients are also burnt up better.

USA: we grew so big

- Fully two-thirds of U.S. adults are officially overweight, and about half of those have graduated to full-blown obesity.

- Among US kids between 6 and 19 years old, 15% (or 1 in 6) are overweight and another 15% are headed that way.

- The cost of obesity-related medical care amounts to 117 billion dollars a year!

Europeans are getting rounder

In the European Union, between 10% and 20% of men and 10% and 25% of women are obese, according to a survey carried out by *the European Association for the Study of Obesity*.

8% of the healthcare costs in the E.U. – about 42 billion euros – go toward the treatment of obesity-related illnesses.

England: Around two-thirds of the English are overweight or obese, with obesity up almost 400% in the last 25 years.

France: Some 32% of the population are overweight and 11% are obese. 18% of children between 6 and 9 are overweight and 3.8% are obese – almost four times as many as in 1960.

Germany: Two-thirds of the male population and about half of the female population are overweight or obese. About 8% of children and teenagers suffer from obesity.

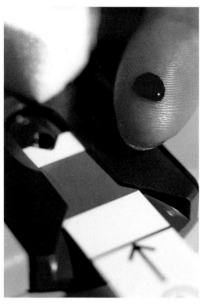

A galloping epidemic: diabetes

In 1995, there were 135 million Type 2 diabetics in the world. Twice that number are predicted in 2015. Simultaneously with obesity, diabetes is increasing vastly, to the extent that we find ourselves in an unprecedented epidemic situation. Could the XXL syndrome be partly responsible for this scourge?

Non-insulin-dependent (NID) diabetes, known as Type 2 diabetes, is a serious disease because of its complications. It sets in very slowly and for this reason occurs late, as a general rule at an age of more than 50. Diabetes is the result of sugar metabolism getting out of order and is defined by fasting glycemia exceeding **1,26 g/l**.

The XXL syndrome promotes increased glycemia

1- In the intestine, excess salt activates glucose assimilation.

The glucose molecule is transported into the intestinal cell through a channel protein. Each glucose molecule is accompanied by two sodium ions. This co-transport is the more efficient because the salt and the glucose are present simultaneously. Indeed, the salt increases the channel protein's affinity for glucose. Thus, the more sodium there is in the intestine, the more glucose molecules are absorbed and the more will be found in the blood.

2- The swollen cells no longer capture blood glucose

Metabolic blockage affects the metabolism of all the nutrients that are co-transported by the sodium. First and foremost: glucose. Too much salt in our food means too much glucose and sodium in our cells. For lack of potassium, since the Na/K pump cannot manage to expel the sodium, the cells become engorged with water. With their metabolism blocked, they cease to capture blood glucose. Glycemia remains high.

When there is a shortage of potassium, glucose intolerance appears

Researchers have subjected healthy people to a low-potassium diet. After a week, the total body potassium concentration had decreased greatly. After a high-glucose test meal, the amount of glucose metabolised was distinctly lower than that measured when body potassium concentration was normal. Part of the glucose remained in the blood.[15]

The chemical damage done by glucose

The major complication in diabetes comes from glycation of the hemoglobin in the red blood cells. Excess blood glucose promotes a chemical reaction: glucose fixation on the hemoglobin in the red blood cells, which is termed glycation. The red blood cells become less supple and this leads to microcirculation disorders in the capillaries, notably in the retina, the kidneys and the extremities. Glycation may also occur in the insulin, which in turn becomes inactive. This would partly explain insulin resistance.

The diuretics test

The hypothesis according to which glucose intolerance derives from a shortage of potassium is supported by studies on diuretics. These medicines, by promoting water elimination with the urine, lead to potassium losses and... glucose intolerance. And the effect is reversible. When potassium is taken at the same time as diuretics, this intolerance can partly be corrected.[16]

Too much salt promotes resistance to insulin

This has been demonstrated in man[17] and by several experiments conducted on animals. Researchers have thus demonstrated that if rats are given a high-salt diet, after several weeks they display resistance to insulin (a decrease in insulin's action, which normally orders the cells to capture glucose). The interesting thing is that if potassium is added to the diet, resistance to insulin is lessened in the muscles, the liver and the entire body. The researchers concluded that "potassium supplementation could be an effective means of preventing resistance to insulin".[18, 19, 20]

A concatenation of nervous disorders

Of all our tissues, the nervous system is the most sensitive to the working of the Na/K pump since it is the site of the nervous impulse which is transmitted through the movements of sodium and potassium ions through channels in the plasma membrane.

When potassium falls, so does morale

A potassium deficiency is often combined with sadness or mood swings and a feeling of not being well. In depressives, the potassium concentration in the cells is lower than in people in good mental health. Similarly, low brain potassium levels have been found after suicide.[23]

It was on squid neurons that Holding and Huxley, between 1936 and 1952, carried out important research into potassium channels and were thus able to demonstrate that the nervous system only functions because of the Na/K pump. It can thus be understood that the consequences of the XXL syndrome for the nervous system can be catastrophic.

The nerve impulse does not amount merely to electrical impulses that propagate throughout the body. In some places, in order to continue on their way, the electrical signals are converted into chemical signals, then converted back into electrical impulses. This is what happens in the brain between two neurons. These cells need chemical messengers (neurotransmitters) to communicate, because they are not in contact with one another but are separated by a small space called a synapse. Any Na/K pump dysfunction affects neurotransmission and causes anxiety- and depression-type disorders, and even behavioural disorders.

Two neurotransmission abnormalities: depression and bipolar syndrome

These disorders appear according to the degree of impairment of the functioning of the Na/K pump. If the pump is only moderately affected, membrane excitability increases, as does the emission of chemical messengers. This is then reflected by manic-depressive or bipolar disorders[21]. At the next stage up (Na/K pump severely inhibited), the transmission of electrical signals is affected and is accompanied by a decrease in the emission of neurotransmitters that may give rise to depression[22]. When this decrease involves serotonin, dopamine or noradrenaline, which are the principal good mood mediators, sadness and pessimism predominate.

It is interesting to note that bipolar disorders are at present treated with lithium, a metal that belongs to the same chemical family as potassium and sodium and that acts like potassium by activating the Na/K pump. The problem with lithium is that it is difficult to handle since the toxic dose is very close to the therapeutic dose. We believe that lithium could easily be replaced by potassium in all these nervous illnesses where it is used.

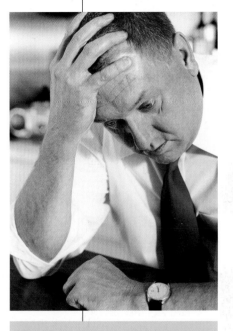

The bipolar syndrome

This disorder is characterised by alternating manic and depressive episodes. Mania, in the psychiatric sense, is the exact reverse of melancholia. The term mania has nothing to do with the customary meaning of the word. Just as melancholia is sad and sombre, so mania is festive. A manic person thinks he is the best, the handsomest, the most intelligent, the richest, the strongest. Patients in a manic state are characterised by their expansiveness, their quicker thinking and reduced sleep.

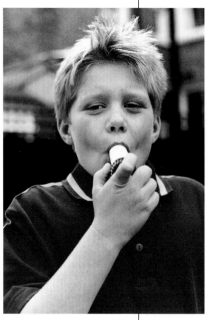

Respiratory tracts exposed to asthma

The XXL syndrome leads to weakness of the respiratory tract, thus making people more liable to asthma.

In a healthy person, the bronchi remain open enough to allow free, comfortable inspiration and expiration, requiring no particular effort. In a person suffering from the XXL syndrome, the respiratory tract is easily irritated. The mechanical properties of the airways are modified because of the slowing of the Na/K pump. The contractility of the smooth muscle tissue of the bronchi is impaired. At the next stage above, an asthma attack occurs. The metabolic blockage of the cells leads to swelling of the walls of the bronchi, causing narrowing of the respiratory tract and reducing the flow of air inspired and expired. Breathing becomes laboured. The person then feels tightness of the chest and distressing breathlessness.

Salt accused

An English doctor, Peter Burney, in a study conducted in 1987, was the first to implicate salt intake by asthmatics, particularly where the outcome was fatal. This research was continued and confirmed by other teams, showing that salt intake promoted bronchial hyperreactivity and aggravated asthma attacks.[24]

The incidence of asthma is therefore higher in people with a high salt intake, whether child or adult, man or woman, city dweller or countryman.

More important, when salt intake by asthmatics is reduced from 10 g to 5 g per day, an improvement in the symptoms is noted. Attacks are less frequent. The patients take less medication.

Can potassium be beneficial?

A study carried out in Sweden suggests that this is the case. Thirty-five asthmatics followed a vegetarian diet for a year: **fresh** fruit and vegetables ad libitum, no meat or milk or eggs, no prepared dishes. No added **salt** or sugar. Their diet was thus high in potassium and low in sodium. At the end of the study, 92% of the participants recognised that their asthma had greatly improved[25]. Another study carried out in England on children confirmed this good effect.

A plant that is useful to asthmatics:
Desmodium adscendens

This plant is currently used in Ghana to treat asthma attacks. Researchers have analysed its different constituents and studied their mode of action. They discovered that this plant contains saponins (soya saponins) which are powerful potassium channel activators (the most effective known to date). By promoting potassium exchanges on either side of the cell membrane, these molecules promote relaxation of the smooth muscle tissue of the bronchi and facilitate breathing. Such compounds are also found in soya (soya saponins) which moreover contains large quantities of them, much more than *Desmodium*.

More and more asthmatics

Known since ancient times, asthma is undergoing a worrying increase. According to the WHO, the number of asthmatics has been increasing by 50% every ten years for the past 30 years. 150 million people are thought to be affected worldwide, including 14 million in the USA and about 15 million in Europe. Asthma affects all age groups, but often develops during childhood. There is a parallel between the rise of asthma in the world, ever-increasing salt intake and potassium deficiency. This is indeed the very heart of the XXL Syndrome.

It is estimated that at world level, asthma-related costs exceed the costs of tuberculosis and AIDS together.

Salt and cancer: the evidence

Salt is heavily implicated in digestive diseases. Excess salt means excess sodium but also excess chlorine (10 g of salt contain 4 g of sodium and 6 g of chlorine), and chlorine is just as dangerous as sodium.

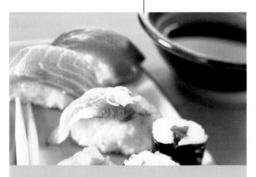

Salt fish and soya sauce: hello trouble!

In South-East Asia, the incidence of stomach cancer varies considerably from one country to another. Thus there is five times more cancer in Vietnam than in Thailand. Researchers wanted to know what, in their lifestyles, could account for such a wide difference. At the end of their study, the risk factor at the top of the list was high salt intake. It would seem to increase the risk of stomach cancer by 80%.[28]

Chlorine is excreted in the gastric mucosa to form hydrochloric acid in the stomach. It is this acid that enables us to digest food. Unfortunately, an excess of chlorine leads to an accumulation of hydrochloric acid. The too-acid gastric juices damage the mucosa that protects the stomach. This opens the door to ulcers and later to stomach cancer.

Stomach cancer and salt: a strong correlation

The INTERSALT[26] study showed that stomach cancer was very common in populations who preserved their foodstuffs in salt. These stomach cancers are often accompanied by strokes, which are connected with excessive salt intake, as we have already seen. In those same countries, when the incidence of vascular accidents decreases due to better treatment of hypertension, the incidence of stomach cancers does not decrease.

Fruit and vegetables provide protection

Potassium has not been studied as a protective factor against cancer and stomach ulcers, as it has in other salt-related illnesses, but it is known that a diet high in fruit and vegetables, and thus in potassium, gives protection against degenerative diseases of the digestive tract.

A large-scale Swedish study showed an inverse relationship between fruit and vegetable consumption and the incidence of stomach cancer. Eleven thousand twins (same genotype, therefore comparable innate risks) were tracked for 35 years: at the end of this very long study, it was found that the risk of stomach cancer was in inverse ratio to fruit and vegetable consumption. The ones who ate little fruit and vegetables were five times more at risk of developing a digestive cancer[27]. Is the whole benefit attributable to potassium alone? Maybe not, because account may also be taken of the effects of vitamin C and lycopene, an anti-cancer substance found in particular in tomatoes, but this detracts nothing from potassium's merits because its rôle is of such capital importance in many cellular phenomena.

Cancer prevention

In his book: *"Naissance de la médecine prédictive"* (*"The Birth of Predictive Medicine"*), Jacques Ruffié[30] writes that cancer cases in developed countries have increased due to changes in diet: fewer cereals and green vegetables, more steak/chips. He also writes that cancers decrease in line with the consumption of fruit and vegetables high in antioxidant vitamins. In fact, he forgets that vegetables and fruit are above all very high in potassium. It is in fact potassium, by re-equilibrating our cell metabolism, that has the major responsibility for preventing cancer.

Chlorine: a carcinogen

Chlorine is very widely used in the water treatment industry to ensure good microbiological quality. But it gives rise to compounds that are suspected, in the long term, of promoting certain types of cancers, particularly cancer of the bladder.

Spanish researchers have just analysed the results of 8 epidemiological studies. They conclude that people who, for several decades, drink water treated with chlorinated compounds, see their risk of cancer of the bladder, compared with other people, increase by 20-30% on average. In men this increase can be as high as 40%.[28]

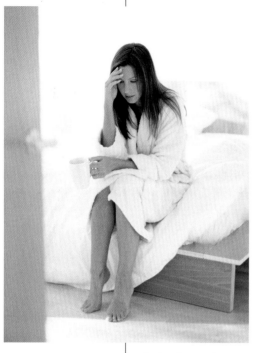

Fatigue and lack of energy: remember potassium

When the cells are in a state of metabolic blockage, energy disappears. Check your potassium level!

If a large part of your cells are no longer assimilating enough nutrients because of an excess of sodium and a lack of potassium, how can they be in good shape and provide the energy the body needs to move and react? It would be a real achievement. When the XXL syndrome sets in, the muscle cells contract badly, the nerve cells are flat out, you feel tired, listless, empty. A wave of weariness engulfs you.

Chronic fatigue syndrome: a matter of potassium

A shortage of potassium is the common denominator in a good number of fatigue situations. Recently, a study showed that people suffering from chronic fatigue syndrome have a considerably lower total body potassium concentration (up to 10% lower) than people who are in good form[31]. Blood potassium levels being normal, this reduced concentration essentially affects the intracellular medium. Remember that 90% of potassium is inside the cells, especially muscle (40% of total potassium), liver and red blood cells. According to the same researchers, by restoring the potassium status, the patients' energy level is improved. This was what they found when they gave these people medication enabling them to retain potassium (spironolactone, a potassium-sparing sodium diuretic).

Sportspeople, watch your potassium closely!

Potassium is absolutely decisive in sports performance, recovery and muscle development. It plays a basic part in muscle excitability and contractile capacity. These two parameters depend on the Na/K pump being in good working order. If this pump shows any signs of weakness (XXL syndrome), excitability is affected and muscular strength decreases. For sportspeople, it cannot be denied that this has repercussions on performance. Consequently, before any sustained physical effort, it is important for sportspeople to ensure that their potassium intake is sufficient.

Chronic fatigue syndrome, what's that?

This illness was really identified in 1988 and it is estimated that 2% of people who complain of chronic fatigue are suffering from it. They feel exhausted in the face of the very ordinary tasks of day-to-day life. The sufferer is not depressive. The joy of living is there and they would love to do all sorts of things but the slightest activity leaves them exhausted for several days.

To cure this illness, take potassium and vegetable Na/K channel activators (*see p.63*).

It's the sodium-potassium pump that keeps us going!

When Na/K pump activity is reduced through ouabain, a molecule capable of binding to these pumps, preventing them from functioning, muscular fatigue appears sooner. Conversely, it is deferred when the pumps are stimulated[32]. Conclusion: if you want to feel full of beans, top up with potassium!

Osteoporosis and brittle bones: a matter of pH

What is pH?

It is a Swedish chemist, Arrhenius, who discovered a method of calculating the acidity or basicity of an aqueous solution.

When you put an acid into solution, e.g. HCl, hydrochloric acid, that acid splits into ions: Cl^- and H^+.

On the other hand, when you put basic products in solution, e.g. caustic soda NaOH, Na^+ and OH^- ions form. OH- is responsible for basicity and, by combining with H+, forms water: $OH^- + H^+ = H2O$.
• If there is as much H^+ as OH^-, the solution is neither acid, nor basic, it is neutral.
• The more H^+ ions there are in solution, the more acid the solution becomes. Arrhenius' scale goes from 0 to 14. The lower the pH, the more acid the solution:
  - from 0 to 7, the number of H^+ ions decreases down to 0
  - at 7, the solution is neutral
  - then from 7 to 14, the solution becomes more and more basic.

The ideal pH for life is 7.2. It is slightly basic. If you become acid, you will have health problems.

Many factors promote the onset of osteoporosis: lack of physical activity, smoking, alcohol, the menopause. But excess sodium and potassium deficiency make a very large contribution. The XXL syndrome continues to strike…

A matter of pH

For the cells to function properly, intracellular pH must be maintained within narrow limits (6.8 – 7.2). It is regulated by membrane ion exchanges and essentially by a particular exchanger, the Na^+/H^+ pump. This pump counters acidification of the intracellular medium: as it lets in an Na^+ ion it expels an H^+ proton. Without this pump, the cell would accumulate protons and the pH would fall considerably (down to 6). Only the thing is this: its working depends directly, from an energy point of view, on the working of the Na/K pump. If the Na/K pump is working in slow motion, the Na/H pump is inevitably less efficient. When this maladjustment affects a large number of cells, as is the case with the XXL syndrome, it causes **acidosis**.

The consequence of acidosis: bones become brittle

Potassium is the most important alkalising mineral in the body. When salt is taken in excess, potassium, its cell exchange currency, shows a deficit. The body, in order to restore the acid-base equilibrium, is therefore obliged to call up another alkalising cation, calcium, which it takes from its reserves, i.e. the skeleton. The XXL syndrome promotes bone resorption and makes bones brittle[33].

Potassium banishes the spectre of osteoporosis

Our Paleolithic ancestors had perfectly healthy bones. They ate no salt and above all, they took in nearly three times as much potassium as we do.[34] In our contemporaries, studies show that people who eat enough fruit and vegetables have alkaline urine and better bone density that those who eat little of them[35]. Proof that by increasing potassium intake to the detriment of sodium, bone health is improved, has recently been provided by the American DASH study. The researchers asked 186 adults to modulate their sodium intake: 3.5 g/day for one month then 2.3 g/day the following month and finally 1.2 g/day; half of these people were also following the DASH diet. Remember that this diet is high in fruit and vegetables and lightened dairy products, therefore high in potassium, magnesium and calcium. By measuring different bone metabolism parameters, the researchers concluded that the DASH diet significantly reduced bone resorption, that reducing salt intake decreased urinary calcium elimination and that these two measures had complementary beneficial effects on bone health.[36]

Salt, the calcium thief

The more salt is absorbed, the more calcium is eliminated in the urine: for every 6 g of salt absorbed, 40 mg of calcium are eliminated. It has thus been calculated that a postmenopausal woman who reduced her salt intake from 10 to 5 g per day would improve her bone density in the same proportion as if she increased her calcium intake by 1000 mg[38]. But girls, too, must be wary of salt. When they eat salty food, they eliminate more calcium and thus start using up their bone stock very early. You have to start preparing to have strong bones right from childhood.[39]

Stronger bones due to potassium supplementation

In postmenopausal women, potassium bicarbonate supplementation improves the calcium-phosphorus balance, increases bone turnover and slows bone resorption. A study by Sebastian A[37] has demonstrated how useful potassium bicarbonate is.

All that salt, it ages you

Potassium is the most important mineral in the body. It is vital to our cells, just as vital as water and air. But unlike these two elements, there is no warning when we are short of it with the result that the damage starts insidiously, one thing leads to another and we end up ageing prematurely.

Potassium against urine leakages

Taking all ages together, one-third of women experience urine leakages, more often than not occasional. After 65, it happens to one woman out of two. With advancing age, the bladder's ability to distend decreases and its involuntary contractions become more frequent, which promotes urinary incontinence. By activating the Na/K pump, potassium seems to relax the bladder's muscle fibres and thus lessen the pressing need to urinate. Take potassium supplements for this purpose.

Chronic excess salt and potassium deficiency accelerate ageing.

Researchers have noted a direct relationship between age-related decline and Na/K pump activity[40]: as the years go by, these pumps become less efficient. The cells stop working, one after another, fats and sugar accumulate, essential nutrients are not channelled and used so well. In a word: we grow old. A leitmotif of this book recurs here: as soon as the working of the Na/K pump falters, everything goes wrong. A very clear sign that this pump is not working so well is that with advancing age, it is easier to put on weight and there is a greater tendency to develop Type 2 diabetes.

The body, not exactly like it was before

One of the principal characteristics of ageing is the loss of muscle mass. It begins to become evident from the age of 30 in men, later in women, and the process accelerates under pressure from the XXL syndrome. By promoting acidosis, excess salt and chronic potassium shortage promote loss of muscle tone. The scenario is the same for the skeleton. The XXL syndrome leads to a decrease in bone and muscle stock.

My memory's failing

With advancing age, the nervous system changes. The brain is not irrigated as well as it was. Communication between cells is not as good as it was. The rate of nerve impulse decreases (-10 to –30%) from the age of 50. Similarly, there is a decrease in the number of neurons. And the more of them die, the greater the effect on mnenomic capacity. Thus 8 senior citizens out of 10 complain of memory disorders, lapses that are worsened by the XXL syndrome.

• **The XXL syndrome reduces brain blood flow**. The vessel cells are in direct contact with the sodium-rich blood. In a person suffering from the XXL syndrome, these cells engorge with water and swell. The vessels become rigid, their diameter narrows, irrigation of the brain is not so good.

• **Alzheimer's disease: Na/K pump deficiency?** Alzheimer's disease, whose origin is still unknown, is the result of the presence in the brain of lesions associated with a considerable loss of neurons. The onset of Alzheimer's disease is associated with a decrease in brain blood flow and with lower oxygen and glucose consumption in some areas of the brain. It is these two factors that put researchers on the trail of the Na/K pump and the XXL syndrome. If some neurons work in slow motion and even die, it is highly likely that a pump deficiency is involved. This is the thesis maintained by researchers who have noted a significant reduction in the activity of these pumps in the cerebral cortex of Alzheimer sufferers compared with healthy people of the same age.[41]

> To live a long, healthy life, protect your cells by making a significant reduction in your salt intake and eat more fruit and vegetables, or take a potassium supplement!

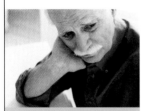

Alzheimer's: the threat

Alzheimer's disease is due to degeneration of neurons involved in memory and mental functions. More often than not, this incurable disease develops into dementia, i.e. physical and mental decline together with a loss of independence. In the majority of cases, the disease develops at around the age of 70. It is estimated that there are about 4.5 million Alzheimer's sufferers in the USA. Experts say there will be more than 13 million patients in 2050!

It is estimated that there are more than 4.7 million Alzheimer's sufferers in Europe. It is worth noting that more women than men are affected (3.5 million against 2.1 million).

HEALTH PROGRAMME

Your health is in your own hands

After this long journey through our cells, their composition, their potassium content and after having taken cognisance of the dangers of excess sodium, we must now get to grips with the problem.

A special mention for Arkocaps

Arkocaps, launched by Arkopharma in 1982, merit a special note. All Arkocaps have an intense effect on the XXL syndrome because all of them contain between 5 and 10% of potassium and all of them also contain more or less flavonoids and saponins. At the time when Arkocaps were launched, the potassium channels had barely been studied and their full importance to our health was not known. Nowadays, twenty years after the launch of Arkocaps, when the potassium channels and potassium are assuming prime importance in medicine, it is easy to imagine that Arkocaps are going to enjoy a new lease of life.

The pharmacology of phytotherapy, or how plants act to improve your health, will have to be reviewed.

What must be done to keep in good health and avoid all the illnesses and annoyances of the XXL syndrome?

• **Rule 1:** avoid taking too much salt in your food by knowing how to spot hidden salt.

• **Rule 2:** improve your potassium level, i.e. eat foods that are high in potassium or take potassium capsules, avoiding potassium chloride if possible because chlorine is as dangerous as sodium.

• **Rule 3:** make the sodium/potassium pump's work easier by having recourse, as prehistoric man did when he lived on wild plants, to plant potassium channel activators. Nowadays, these activators are found in a fair number of medicinal plants.

Survey of potassium channel activators

• Many studies[42] show that **flavonoids** are sodium/potassium pump activators. They promote cell functioning and their vital functions. Now, medicinal plants contain a lot of flavonoids. This is why many of them have pharmacological activity.

For example:
- **hawthorn** in cardiovascular disease,
- **olive tree leaf** for hypertension
- **butcher's broom** for microcirculation and heavy legs problems
- **horse chestnut** against haemorrhoids.

• The second class of substances that activate the potassium channels: **saponins**.

The saponins contained in the plant *Desmodium adscendens* and in soya have shown action on asthma, microcirculation problems and some intestinal illnesses such as irritable bowel syndrome. Thus it is the saponins in **maté** that, by activating the potassium channels, facilitate weight loss. It is also the saponins in **ivy** and **mullein** that, by stimulating those same channels, promote the elimination of bronchial mucus, soothe irritating coughs or improve the symptoms of chonic obstructive bronchopneumopathy (COBP).

• Many other substances, such as **soya isoflavones** associated with soya saponins, also have this property of activating the potassium channels and are used for disorders related to the menopause and a great many other ailments.

> Medicinal plants are the first remedies to use for XXL syndrome illnesses. They all contain potassium and numerous Na/K pump activators: flavonoids, saponins and many other plant compounds.

How to optimise your sodium and potassium intake

Now that you have realised all the benefits, in health terms, that you can derive from a better balance between sodium and potassium, the question arises of how much and how. In other words, what is the optimum potassium /sodium (K/Na) ratio and how can it be achieved?

Return to basics

For thousands of years, man ate foods that never contained much sodium and were always high in potassium. Dr Boyd Eaton (University of Atlanta, Georgia) has devised several prehistoric diet models[43], which have been validated on hunter-gatherers of recent years. In terms of daily intake, a Yanomano Indian in Amazonia, who lives almost exclusively on plants, absorbs 20 to 300 mg of sodium and 3 g or more of potassium. An omnivorous diet such as that of a Kalahari Bushman or a New Guinea Papuan provides between 900 and 1400 mg of sodium without reducing potassium intake, which remains at 3 g.[44]

Dietary supplies of sodium and potassium
in the Upper Paleolithic era and in the present-day USA

Minerals (mg)	Paleolithic age	Present-day USA
Sodium	600	4 000
Potassium	7 000	2 500
Potassium/sodium ratio	12	0,6

The Upper Paleolithic diet is much higher in potassium and much lower in sodium. The dietary K/Na ratio between Paleolithic times and the present day has been reduced by a factor of 20. Now, from a genetic point of view, we are no different from Cro-Magnon man. Nowadays, we are in a completely opposite situation to that of early man, whose kidneys had to retain sodium, which was scarce, and excrete potassium, which was available in abundance.

While it seems difficult to return to prehistoric man's diet, our health would be greatly improved if, by **reducing salt ingestion** and **increasing our potassium intake**, our dietary K/Na ratio were at least equal to 1. According to some experts, the optimum ratio would, in fact, be 5/1. For our Na/K pumps to work properly, for our cells to return to a normal size and recover all their energy, we ought to ingest 5 times more potassium than sodium, in order to achieve a ratio of more than 10/1 inside our cells.[45]

> **It is not necessary to go without salt on your food in order to reduce your risk of cardiovascular disease, diabetes, osteoporosis, to be in good form and age gracefully. It is merely a matter of reducing intake as much as possible and especially, which is easier to do, increasing potassium intake, in order to re-establish the biologically optimum ratio of sodium to potassium.**

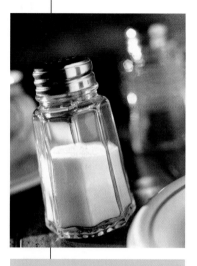

The French and salt

The Inca survey carried out in 1998 and 1999 involved 1985 people over the age of 15 and 1018 children and adolescents. The results show an average salt intake of 8 g/day in adults. Taking the "salt cellar" into account, it can be estimated that according to this survey, the French take in about 10 g of salt per day. In 1994, a survey of the same type had shown lower salt intakes (around 7.5 g/day). This increase in intake is explained by the fact that the French are eating more pizzas, quiches, savoury tarts and other pastries.

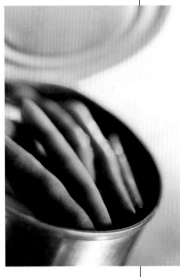

How to take less salt in your food

With a little discernment and a bit of effort, reducing salt intake is within everyone's reach. In the early stages, tell yourself that it's good for your health and in the end, you'll see, you'll do it because you like it.

Reducing salt intake is not as simple as it sounds because it is not the salt cellar on the table that is the trouble, it is the "hidden" salt contained in industrial foods. It accounts for between 70 and 80% of the salt we absorb. An excellent preservative, a flavour enhancer, it improves the taste and appearance of foods. For this reason, it is everywhere, even in unexpected places: chocolate, biscuits, yoghurt, milk desserts, soft drinks, etc. The principal salt-vectoring foods are bread and bakery products, delicatessen products, soups, cheeses, ready meals, pizzas, quiches and savoury tarts, sandwiches, Viennese rolls, seafood, meat and poultry, condiments and sauces.

To take less salt in your food, common sense dictates that you eat fewer high-salt industrial products and give preference to fresh produce, cooked at home, and go easy on the salt.

The surprises in tinned foods

Per 100 g	Potassium (mg)	Sodium (mg)
Raw French beans	243	4
Cooked French beans	240	3
Tinned French beans	107	307

Where is salt hidden?

Salt contained naturally in foods: 10%
Salt added during cooking or at the table: 15%
Salt added during industrial processing: 75

Beware of lightened products

These have literally invaded supermarket shelves. Unfortunately, in order to make these low-fat foods taste nice, salt is added liberally.

A few tricks to reduce salt intake

• Shed the habit of adding salt to everything you eat. At the beginning, the food will seem tasteless, but as time goes on, your taste buds will get used to it. You will rediscover the foods' real taste and with it, the pleasure of eating. What's more, you will then spontaneously shy away from too-salty foods. You just have to follow your instincts.

• Replace salt with other condiments: garlic, parsley, celery, onion, thyme, mixed herbs, pepper. On the other hand, avoid mustard (it has a very high salt content) and many other industrial condiments (meat or chicken stock cubes, packeted sauces, ketchup, ready-made salad dressings). Use high-potassium "salt" (from pharmacies).

• Limit delicatessen products, cooked dishes, preserves, smoked fish, crisps, savoury biscuits, roasted and salted dried oilseeds.

• Rinse tinned vegetables in order to remove as much salt as possible.

• Avoid putting salt in the water used to cook pasta, rice or vegetables.

• Do not get your children used to eating too-salty food because dietary habits are inculcated in childhood and it is difficult to change them once adulthood is reached.

How much sodium do we need?

Theoretically, physiological needs are satisfied with 2 g of salt per day, i.e. 800 mg of sodium. In France and the USA, the health authorities are in agreement in recommending a daily intake of 2.4 g of sodium (i.e. 6 g of salt per day). This is far too much.

The sources of sodium

High-salt foods	Sodium (in mg)
Salami-type sausage (100 g)	1 000-2 000
10 olives (30 g)	600-900
1 portion of quiche Lorraine (130 g)	680
1 slice of smoked ham (40 g)	640
1 slice of boiled ham (40 g)	560
30 g of cereals, 1 pain au chocolat (80 g)	350-400
1 portion of hard cheese (30 g)	330-350
1 portion of roquefort cheese (15 g)	240
1 slice of smoked salmon (20 g)	240
1 slice of white bread (30 g)	150
1/2 tre of milk	220

As the formula of salt is sodium chloride with 40% of sodium and 60% of chloride, 1000 mg of sodium represents 2500 mg of salt.

Potassium for my cells

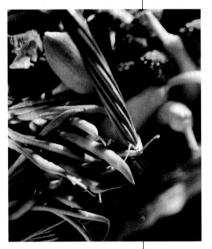

Fruit and vegetables are our main source of potassium. They should take first place in our diet.

How much potassium do we need?

Unlike vitamins, there is no recommended daily allowance for potassium because there are numerous dietary sources. However, in view of the extent of the health problems related to excessive intake of salt and industrial foods, to the detriment of fresh produce, American health services have just published a study report laying down an "adequate intake" of potassium for each age group.[46]

Cooking tips

Avoid blanching your vegetables. Plunging them into boiling water causes their potassium to escape into the cooking water; about 30% of potassium is lost. Eat stir-fried or roasted vegetables. They will retain all their potassium.

Adequate potassium intake in g/day

	Age	Male	Female
Babies	0-6 months	0,4	0,4
Babies	7-12 months	0,7	0,7
Children	1-3 years	3,0	3,0
Children	4-8 years	3,8	3,8
Children	9-13 years	4,5	4,5
Adolescents	14-18 years	4,7	4,7
Adults	19 and over	4,7	4,7
Pregnant women	14-50 years	-	4,7
Nursing mothers	14-50 years	-	5,1

According to the authors, **4.7 g** is the minimum amount of potassium that an adult must ingest every day in order to reduce the risk of chronic disease.

Where can potassium be found?

Dietary sources are many and varied since this mineral is the major constituent in plants and animal cells. Even though meat, dairy products and cereals do contain potassium, overall these foods acidify the body. It is therefore better to increase your vegetable and fruit consumption.

• **Fruit and vegetables** *ad libitum*: 2-4 portions of fruit and 3-5 portions of vegetables per day. The best sources of potassium (per 100 kcal) are leafy green vegetables (spinach, lettuce), tomatoes, cucumber, courgettes, aubergines, pumpkins and root vegetables (carrots, radishes, turnips).

• **Rediscover almonds, hazels and other nuts.** High in fibre, they contain good fatty acids (unsaturated fatty acids) and are an excellent source of potassium.

• **Remember to use fruit as snacks more often, or, for die-hards, fruit juice,** even though it contains less potassium (use really ripe fruit, put it through the blender and drink immediately). When buying, give preference to 100% pure fruit juices with no added sugar.

Potassium content (mg/100 g)

Fats	0
Sugar	0
Egg	128
White bread	132
Milk	150
Raspberries, blackberries, peaches	220
Kiwi fruit, cherries, gooseberries, grapes	280
Wholemeal bread	350
Artichokes	350
Beef	370
Apricots, coconut	380
Pork	390
Chocolate	400
Fish	400
Mushrooms	420
Turkey	490
Veal	500
Fresh avocado pear	522
Fresh spinach	529
Baked potatoes	536
Raw black radish	554
Banana	600
Fresh chervil	600
Dates	670
Walnuts	690
Dried lentils	700
Roasted peanuts	710
Almonds	800
Dried prunes	950
Dried bananas	1150
Dried haricot beans	1450
Dried apricots	1520
Cocoa powder	1920
Red peppers	2000
Wine (mg/litre)	*780*

Potassium as salt or in capsules

Who should take a potassium supplement?

Apart from prevention of cardiovascular and bone diseases, there are some special situations requiring potassium supplementation. Are you taking an anti-hypertensive drug? Ask your doctor whether you should be put on a potassium supplement: some antihypertensives (not all) increase potassium elimination. Potassium supplements are recommended for people on long-term corticosteroids or antibiotics (penicillin). Athletes and manual workers may also benefit from supplements.

Mineral waters

Most mineral waters contain more sodium than potassium. Sodium is more soluble than potassium in the run-off waters that constitute the soil water which will emerge as natural or artificial springs. Only FIUGGI water, in the Italian town of Fiuggi, contains more potassium than sodium. It would be useful for recombined mineral waters, such as Coca Cola's Dasani, to be enriched with potassium, which would make them better for our health.

If you have trouble obeying the rule about 5 portions of fruit and vegetables per day, there are potassium supplements that make it possible to top up the intake.

Exchange your table salt for a potassium salt

Potassium salt is a dietetic salt obtainable at pharmacies that is used like ordinary salt. High in potassium (30%), it provides very little sodium (8%) while retaining the salty taste of traditional salt. It should be noted that in this salt, the potassium is bound to the bicarbonate, the form in which potassium is found in vegetables, and not to the chloride (of which there is little in fruit and vegetables).

Potassium supplements

When the diet does not provide adequate amounts of potassium, supplementation can be used. Capsules containing potassium in the form of bicarbonate are available at pharmacies. The recommended dosage is 2 capsules per day. In healthy people, a higher dietary potassium intake than the recommended daily allowance is not dangerous because the excess potassium is simply eliminated in the urine. The supplements are therefore safe.

Watch your magnesium

To correct a potassium deficiency, it is essential to have a satisfactory magnesium status. Without magnesium, the cells cannot retain potassium.

Magnesium is the second intracellular cation in importance. Like potassium, it is abundant in all vegetables. Magnesium plays a key part in membrane ion equilibrium. It is necessary for the working of the Na/K pump because it allows it to be supplied with energy (ATP fixation to the enzyme).

Magnesium deficiency is common

All magnesium is supplied by the diet. But present-day diet is far from covering requirements. According to the SU.VI.MAX study conducted in France on 5000 people, 77% of women and 72% of men have a magnesium supply lower than the recommended daily intake (recommended daily allowance: adult women: 360 mg, adult men: 420 mg).

There are several reasons for these deficiencies. The present-day diet comprises many processed foods, to the detriment of vegetable produce. Moreover, stress engenders physiological mechanisms that consume a great deal of magnesium.

Sources of magnesium

Fruit and vegetables
(the prize goes to cashew nuts, 252 mg of magnesium per 100 g).

Magnesium carbonate capsules,
sold at pharmacies
or **dolomite capsules**
(double calcium and magnesium carbonate).

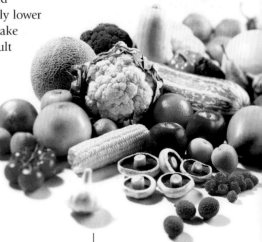

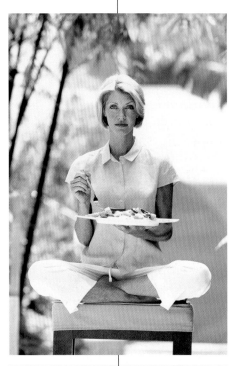

Acid-base: a crucial equilibrium

Potassium is beneficial to the body's acid-base equilibrium but everything depends on the ions that accompany it.

The diet supplies hydrogen (acid) or bicarbonate (basic) ions. According to whether the former predominate or not, the blood is more or less acid. Excess acidity in the blood may increase the risk of osteoporosis (*read p. 58*), diabetes, atherosclerosis, hypertension and some cancers.

Seek bicarbonate

The acidifying foods are meat, milk, cheese and cereals. Nowadays our diet is broadly acid because animal proteins and cereals play a large part in it but also and especially because we eat too few alkalising foods capable of neutralising this acid content. What are these beneficial alkalising foods? High-potassium fruit and vegetables, because the potassium they contain is in the form of bicarbonate or citrate. While the diet in Paleolithic times, compared with ours,

Seeking to increase potassium intake counters the acid-base imbalance induced by our modern diet. So head for fruit and vegetables that provide bicarbonates and give preference to a potassium salt or a potassium supplement in bicarbonate form.

comprised a high proportion of animal proteins (35% or even more), this diet was nonetheless broadly basic because the amount of vegetables, roots and nuts that early man ate was also far higher.

It is interesting to note that in plants, potassium is rarely bound to the chloride. Potassium chloride (KCl), found in some diet salts and in most potassium supplements, does not have the "antacid" properties of potassium bicarbonate. It is therefore less useful. Moreover, as we have already seen on pp. 54-55, chlorine is just as dangerous to health as sodium (Na).

Three consequences of acid-base imbalance

Due to our dietary errors, we are more often than not in a state of acid-base imbalance, with a tendency to be more acid than normal. This acidity has important repercussions on our health.

• It promotes osteoporosis. To restore the acid-base equilibrium, our body draws on the calcium in the skeleton. This is how we become decalcified. Osteoporosis ensues. Taking potassium bicarbonate, by combating acidity, makes it possible to avoid the bones becoming brittle.

• It promotes the growth of yeast in the intestine and, in women, in the vagina. This is candidosis, so common in the USA. The remedy: basify by taking potassium bicarbonate, eat plenty of vegetables and fruit and avoid acidifying foods such as meat and cheese.

• Many clinical trials have shown that acidification of the blood promotes inflammation of the airways and asthmatic reactions[47]. Excess sodium promotes acidification, whereas excess potassium combats acidification. We have explained in this book that potassium and potassium channel activators (saponins, polyphenols) expel sodium from our cells and basify the blood. This is why soya saponins are a great remedy for asthma.

Other benefactors: omega-3 fatty acids

In a book that we published 15 years ago: *La peau de la vie (The skin of life)*, we explained that omega-3 polyunsaturated fatty acids play a crucial part in the body. They make our cell membranes more fluid. Now, this fluidity is a necessity for our cells and, *inter alia*, for the Na/K pump.

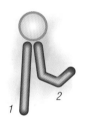

Phospholipids have two fatty acids at 1 and 2. At 1, the fatty acid is always saturated, it is straight and rigid. At 2, it is saturated or unsaturated according to the fatty acids that we consume.

These fatty acids form part of the composition of the membranes of all our cells and their presence is decisive for the latter's fluidity. Our cell membranes are made up of phospholipids, also called lecithin. The more omega-3 there is in these phospholipids, the more fluid our membranes are.

Phospholipids consisting of saturated fatty acids form a dense, rigid membrane structure. Conversely, phospholipids consisting of polyunsaturated fatty acids form a fluid, supple structure.

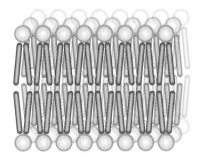

Straight fatty acids = rigid membrane
= **LITTLE CELLULAR EXCHANGE**

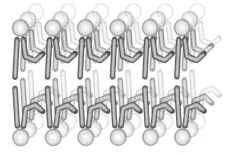

Curved fatty acids = fluid membrane
= **EASY CELLULAR EXCHANGES**

Membrane fluidity facilitates the task of the Na/K pump

We have seen that the Na/K pump is a membrane protein which, after performing contortions, expels three sodium ions from the cell and brings in two potassium ions. Fluid membranes facilitate this pump's task and in general make all cellular exchanges easier. The cells are better able to assimilate nutrients and better able to evacuate their waste. This leads to a concatenation of events.

• Cholesterol will penetrate further into the membranes to make them rigid and will no longer be in the blood, where it risked becoming oxidised.

• When the membranes of the muscle cells are fluid, the red blood cells circulate more easily and blood pressure decreases.

• In the brain, membrane fluidity promotes exchanges between neurons. The memory performs better and exchanges are more intense, promoting brain activity.

Where to find omega-3 fatty acids

Omega-3 fatty acids are found in walnuts, and in rapeseed, soya and walnut oils. But above all in fish, and particularly in fatty fish such as mackerel, salmon, sardines, herrings, trout (tuna contains some as well but it provides too much mercury to be eaten regularly). Tinned salmon, generally wild, is also an excellent source, whereas fresh Atlantic salmon is a farmed fish which, according to a French study published in 1999, supplies ten times less. There is very little omega-3 in meat. Finally, fish oil capsules are available at pharmacies.

Omega-3: benefits to our health

- omega-3 fatty acids are essential to the proper development of the retina and the brain in foetuses and new-born babies;

- they lower the triglyceride level when it is too high;

- they prevent cardiovascular disease and some types of cancer (breast, colon, prostate);

- they have anti-inflammatory properties;

- they reduce the risk of nervous depression by promoting the circulation of the nerve impulse.

Your health regimen

In order to help you to correct the sodium-potassium imbalance in your diet, here is a summary of the foods to which to give preference and those that are best avoided. Go shopping!

Type of food	Give preference to:	Avoid:
Meat	- Game, poultry (chicken, duck, guinea fowl, turkey, goose...without the skin), veal, beef, lamb, rabbit, pork. - Give preference to lean cuts	- Fatty cuts - Pre-packed industrial delicatessen products - Hamburgers - Rillettes, pâté, sausages, salami-type sausage, merguez, andouillettes,lardons, etc.
Seafood	- All fish, giving preference to fatty fish. - In moderation: shellfish, crustaceans.	- Tinned fish in oil (too much salt). - Fish roe (again, too much salt) - Breaded or fried fish - Smoked fish - Frozen fish gratin
Eggs	- Hard boiled, fried, soft boiled, scrambled, omelettes	- Industrial omelettes - Jellied eggs
Vegetables & fruit	- All fresh or frozen vegetables - All fresh fruit - Jacket potatoes - All legumes: lentils, peas, chickpeas, haricot or red kidney beans, broad beans, soyabeans - Almonds, walnuts, peanuts, hazel nuts, cashew nuts, unsalted pistacchio nuts	- Tinned vegetables, packet or tinned soups - Fruit in syrup - Freeze-dried mash, gratin dauphinois and hash Frozen shepherd's pie, crisps - Tinned cassoulet, tinned lentils with sausages, frozen chili con carne - Roasted salted nuts (cocktail nibbles)

Type of food	Give preference to	Avoid
Cereals	- Wholemeal bread, rye bread - Brown rice, wild rice, Basmati rice - Wholemeal and brown pasta - Sugar-free muesli, oat flakes	- White bread, crumby bread, biscottes - Quick white rice, frozen pre-cooked rice - Quick pasta - Cornflakes and all puffed and sweetened breakfast cereals - Viennese rolls, pastries and sweetened industrial biscuits - Cocktail biscuits - Pizzas, quiches, savoury tarts
Dairy products	- Natural yoghurt, cream cheese	- Processed cheese - Sweetened yoghurt and other milk desserts - Chocolate milk shakes
Fats, seasoning and assaisonnement et condiments	- Olive, rapeseed, walnut and soya oil - Rapeseed margarine - Garlic, onions, shallots, parsley, basil, tarragon, chives, thyme, rosemary, laurel, etc. .	- Slightly salted butter, crème fraîche - Solid fats for frying - Stock cubes, packet sauces, nuoc mâm, Kikkoman soy sauce (Teryaki) - Mustard, ketchup - Ready-made vinaigrette sauce - Gherkins
Drinks	- Mineral water - Fresh fruit juice or 100% pure juice free from added sugar - Herbal teas - Wine (1-2 glasses per day)	- Some kinds of aerated water (read the label) - Tomato juice - Soft drinks - In moderation: alcohol, coffee, tea

Hypertension

Less salt, more potassium: why?

If you reduce the salt in your food, the volume of the artery cells decreases. The arteries are more supple and offer less resistance to the flow of blood. Blood pressure falls. And it falls even further if, at the same time, potassium intake is increased (*read p. 33*).

My dietary advice

• Reducing excess weight is an essential step.

• The quality of the food is of prime importance, so follow the health regimen (*pp. 76-77*) to the letter!

• Excessive alcohol intake is held responsible for about 10% of hypertension. Limit yourself to a maximum of two glasses of red wine per day (one glass for women). Beyond that level, drinking alcohol is harmful.

• Moderate but regular and prolonged physical exercise 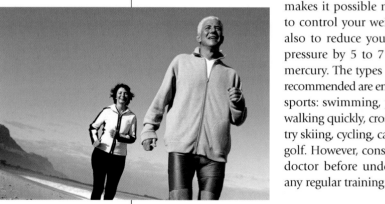 makes it possible not only to control your weight but also to reduce your blood pressure by 5 to 7 mm of mercury. The types of sport recommended are endurance sports: swimming, jogging, walking quickly, cross-country skiing, cycling, canoeing, golf. However, consult your doctor before undertaking any regular training.

My phytotherapeutic advice

The active part of the **olive tree** is its leaf. It is traditionally used by meridional populations to obtain diuretic and hypotensive effects. It also has anti-arrhythmic and coronary artery dilating properties. Olive tree leaf is particularly indicated for moderate hypertension, as a curative treatment and to prevent progression to a more severe form of hypertension with cardiovascular repercussions.

Garlic acts on the blood platelets by decreasing their aggregation capacity. It thus fluidifies the blood, accelerating blood circulation and combating hypertension. It is olive tree leaf's essential complement.

Hawthorn is a friend to the heart. It regulates cardiac rhythm and acts more widely on the whole of the circulatory system. It increases coronary blood flow and reduces blood pressure.

Pitfalls to avoid

• Stress tends to make blood pressure rise. So stay cool, either by avoiding stressful situations or by learning how to overcome them. Managing stress and relaxing can be learnt!

• Daily consumption of liquorice or products containing it can cause or worsen hypertension.

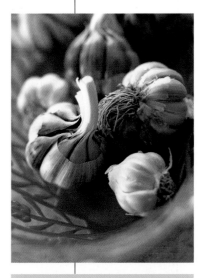

Potassium for the prevention of strokes

Epidemiological studies, like the one carried out by Harvard University that tracked 43,000 Americans, suggest that people whose potassium intake is high (whether it be dietary potassium or nutritional supplements) are at less risk of a stroke. Supplements could also prevent heart attacks.

Diabetes (TYPE 2)

What is the glycemic index?

The GI measures a food's ability to raise glycemia. This value is pegged to the same quantity of a reference food, in the case in point glucose or white bread. For example, compared with white bread (GI 100), a natural yoghurt has a GI of 62, which is fairly low, whereas a chocolate bar has a GI of 80, which is rather high.

SOKOJA DIABETES

Sokoja Diabetes is a range of high-protein packet soups containing plant extracts, notably including tulsi. It is useful to replace the midday meal with a packet of Sokoja Diabetes and a piece of fruit. You will lose weight and regularise your carbohydrate metabolism.

Less salt, more potassium: why?

By reducing salt in your food and increasing your potassium intake, the amount of glucose absorbed in the intestine is reduced and sensitivity to insulin is improved, which makes it easier to regulate glycemia (*read p. 21 & p. 48*).

My dietary advice

First and above all, control your weight, then equilibrate glycemia to the best of your ability both by **physical activity** and **dietetics**.

Diabetics must split up their meals to "smooth out" their blood glucose level (glycemia) as much as possible.

To slow sugar absorption, you must:
• know which carbohydrates have a low glycemic index and choose them,
• reduce the overall amount of sugar consumed,
• and above all increase your fibre intake.

To achieve this fibre intake but also to increase vitamin and mineral intake, it is enough to eat cooked and/or raw vegetables at the two main meals, as well as fruit at least once a day, preferably as a snack.

Two protein-based meals must be taken every day:
• lunch will be the meal of choice for good animal protein (meat, poultry or fish);
• the morning or evening meal will include a different

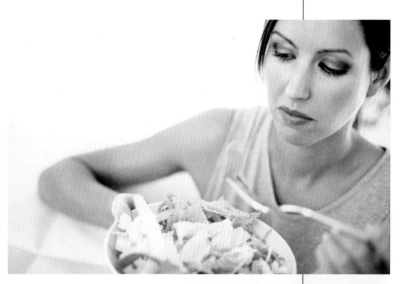

protein, possibly a milk or vegetable protein. Reducing saturated fats (red meat, delicatessen products and milk fats) as much as possible, and giving preference to good quality vegetable oils is another essential aim in order to avoid diabetic complications as far as possible.

And practice a sport of some kind every day (30 minutes a day is better than 2 hours on Sunday!)

Dietary supplements

Omega-3 fatty acids: derived from fish oils, these fatty acids have proved their efficacy in the prevention of cardiovascular disease. Moreover, they increase cell sensitivity to insulin and consequently improve sugar metabolism.

Chromium: this trace element plays an important part in sugar utilisation. It stimulates the insulin receptors, enabling the hormone to exert a better action.

Antioxidants: zinc, selenium and vitamin E have shown their good effects on glycemia and glycosylated hemoglobin levels in long-term supplementation trials.

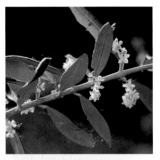

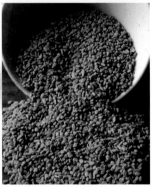

Olive tree leaf and fenugreek

My phytotherapeutic advice

Olive tree leaf in capsule form reduces glycemia and increases diuresis. It also reduces blood pressure, blood LDL-cholesterol (the "bad" one) and triglycerides, and increases the "good" cholesterol fraction. Olive tree leaf thus manages not only glycemia but also the whole of the vascular diathesis, which is weak in diabetics. It is also an antioxidant.

Fenugreek stimulates insulin secretion. A study carried out during the 1990s by a research team in Montpellier isolated an amino acid responsible for fenugreek's hypoglycemic activity: hydroxy-isoleucine.

Indian basil (*Ocimum Sanctum*) or **tulsi** in Hindi, is holy to Indians.. It is used in Type 2 diabetes. Clinical trials carried out in India have shown it to have useful activity in Type 2 diabetes. *Ocimum sanctum* extracts have displayed hypoglycemic activity and a better use of glucose.[48, 49, 50, 51,52]

An extract of Indian basil forms part of the composition of a dietary product for diabetics: Sokoja Diabetes.

Pitfalls to avoid

• Skipping a meal
• Nibbling between authorised food intakes (if you are "dying" for something sweet, increase your physical expenditure).
• Many doctors recommend fructose, preferably white sugar fructose, to their patients. The reason: sweetening power being comparable, fructose does not raise blood sugar. Now, in animals, fructose leads in the long term to the appearance of... diabetes.
• Similarly, beware of sweeteners, because sugar calls to sugar. A diabetic must make every effort to lose his taste for sweet things. He must lose the habit of sweetening his food and drinks, even with sweeteners. Moreover, they very often contain sodium!

Soya saponins

• These are saponins that are abundant in soyabeans but also in haricot beans, broad beans, chick peas and many other legumes. It is soya that has the highest content.

• Soya contains more than eight varieties of soya saponins. They have been studied for more than 100 years and it is thought that they are the most effective potassium channel activator. They have played a big part as a health factor in all peoples who eat, or used to eat, large quantities of legumes in their diet. As they have been used by humans in large quantities for several thousand years, they are absolutely safe.

• A Ghanian plant, Desmodium adscendens, is used in asthma and many illnesses. Its active principles are soya saponins, which are very abundant in this plant.

• Soya saponins should be used in many illnesses characterised by inflammation or when there is an increase in cell volume
- asthma and chronic bronchitis
- irritable bowel syndrome
- hypertension
- type 2 diabetes
- obesity
- illnesses of the nervous system with depressive features
- fatigue and lack of energy

• At the same time as soya saponins, the use of capsules containing potassium in the form of potassium bicarbonate is recommended.

• The dose of soya saponins to use is from 2 to 4 capsules per day

Excess weight

Less salt, more potassium: why?

To lose weight, you have to restore life to cells whose metabolism is slowed by the XXL syndrome. By taking potassium and activating the potassium channels, Na/K pump activity is increased. With the pump working better, sodium is eliminated from the cells, calories are burnt up better and total energy expenditure increases.

4,3,2,1

A plant-based drink, *4,3,2,1 minceur* is proving successful worldwide. This drink causes weight loss, gives energy and makes it possible to recover a normal weight and terrific form. It was devised in accordance with the principles set out in this book, it is high in potassium obtained from plants and it contains a lot of saponins and flavonoids, which are potassium channel activators. All these constituents together get cell metabolism going again, eliminate the sodium that lodges in the cells, promote thermogenesis and thereby weight loss. Moreover, it restores energy. Its success will be long-lasting because it is biologically effective.

My dietary advice

• Follow the health regimen suggested in this book, giving preference to proteins to the detriment of carbohydrates. By eating proteins, you oblige your body to expend energy. Much more energy than is required to digest carbohydrates or lipids. Moreover, they are satisfying. Thus in order to lose weight, the proportion of proteins can be increased to 25% of the calorie ration, giving preference to vegetable proteins. The body then preferentially mobilises fat reserves while the muscle mass is conserved.

• Practice sport and build up your muscles. By increasing your muscle mass, you burn up more energy at rest. Moreover, you also raise the level of fat-burning hormones: testosterone and especially growth hormone.

My phytotherapeutic advice

Maté leaves are high in caffeine and saponins that promote the burning of fats. Moreover, maté slows the progress of the alimentary bolus in the stomach, which makes it an excellent appetite reducer. It also has diuretic properties.

Bitter orange peel *(Citrus aurantium)* contains synephrine, a substance that activates a class of receptors that "give orders" to body fat to burn up in order to supply energy. Citrus aurantium increases thermogenesis, as three studies have shown.

Green tea increases energy expenditure by the combined action of caffeine and a polyphenol (epigallocatechin gallate). Moreover, it stimulates fat oxidation.

Orthosiphon is a powerful drainer of the whole body. Not only does it promote weight loss but in the process it eliminates the waste and toxins that would otherwise clutter up the body, bringing fatigue and demotivation.

Soya saponins (*read p. 83*)

Pitfalls to avoid

• Eschew draconian low-calorie diets. Very frustrating, they attack morale as much as the unwanted kilos. Above all they promote the yo-yo effect: when a normal diet is resumed, the body hastens to reconstitute its reserves

• Do not reduce your dietary fats too much. In the long term (more than a year), studies show that low-fat diets have no effect on bodyweight. The more so because we need fats for our cells to function.

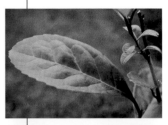

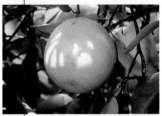

Maté and bitter orange

Need an appetite reducer?

Fucus is a brown alga found abundantly on the rocky coasts of temperate and cold seas in the Northern hemisphere. Because of its mucilaginous structure, fucus rehydrates in the stomach and increase considerably in volume, leading to a feeling of satiety. Fucus acts as a mechanical appetite reducer. Moreover, it improves intestinal transit.

Cholesterol

Less salt, more potassium: why?

By correctly balancing salt and potassium intake, the cells return to their normal size and work better. All forms of metabolism are improved, that of sugar but also that of cholesterol.

A good reason for losing weight

If your cholesterol level is high and you are overweight, you should know that for each kilo of weight loss, your cholesterol will fall by 1%, your LDL-cholesterol by 0.7% and your triglycerides by 2%. As for your HDL-cholesterol, it will rise by 0.2%!

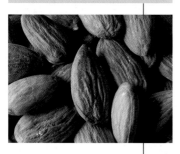

My dietary advice

• Reduce fats high in saturated fatty acids as much as possible: they increase the proportion of bad cholesterol (LDL). More often than not in solid form, they are principally of animal origin: milk fats (butter, cream, cheese), delicatessen products. In order not to commit any dietary errors, put your trust in the health regimen on page 76, but go steady on eggs because they are high in cholesterol (an egg yolk contains 250 mg of it).

• Replace animal proteins with **soya** in all its forms (tofu, milk, yoghurt). Soya proteins check cholesterol production by the liver. They reduce LDL-cholesterol and triglycerides, and increase "good" cholesterol (HDL).

• **Almonds** are worth eating more often. They contain monounsaturated fatty acids similar to those in olive oil, fibres and phytosterols, substances which promote cholesterol elimination in the stools.

• Eat **psyllium** seeds. They are very high in soluble fibres. In the intestines, these fibres form a gel with water to which cholesterol binds, thus preventing its reabsorption.

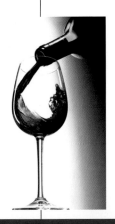

• **Wine** is not forbidden, quite the reverse. It increases the proportion of good cholesterol. As for tea, you can drink as much as you like. The more of it you drink, the lower cholesterol becomes.
• Regular physical activity is strongly recommended. It increases HDL, decreases LDL and keeps triglycerides at bay. Thus the mere fact of leaving your car behind and walking can reduce your cholesterol.

My phytotherapeutic advice

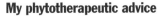

Olive tree leaf is, yet again, the plant for the situation. Olive leaves have hypo-cholesterolemic action (they decrease the level of LDL-cholesterol and increase the level of HDL-cholesterol). A recent study conducted on animals with a high cholesterol level (prediabetic, obese rats) showed that a decoction of olive leaves could reduce this level by 42% while a statin (simvastatin), a synthetic medicine, only managed to reduce it by 32%[53]. No effect was observed on triglycerides or HDL-cholesterol.

Pitfalls to avoid

• Smoking reduces good cholesterol, makes vessel walls brittle and finally dangerously amplifies cardiovascular risk.
• Be careful about coffee; it does indeed contain antioxidants but it is also high in substances that raise cholesterol and blood pressure.

Dietary supplements

Soya lecithin: it promotes solubilisation of fatty acids in the blood, notably cholesterol, and prevents them from being deposited on the artery walls. However, soya lecithin's action does not stop there! High in choline and inositol, it intervenes in hepatic metabolism of fats by increasing the level of good cholesterol and reducing the level of bad cholesterol.

Fish oils: the omega-3 fatty acids EPA and DHA increase the level of HDL and essentially reduce triglycerides.

Vitamin E: this antioxidant vitamin prevents cholesterol from oxidising and blocking the arteries.

Phytosterols: these molecules compete with cholesterol in the intestine, make it less soluble and prevent it from being absorbed. The result: it is eliminated in the stools. In order to note a fall in blood cholesterol, the body has to be supplied with 1 to 2 g of vegetable sterols per day.

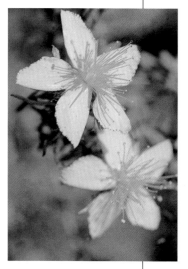

Health target
Depression

Less salt, more potassium: why?

Simply to facilitate cellular exchanges and in particular communication between neurons, by promoting neurotransmitter emission (*read p. 50*).

My dietary advice

• Neurotransmitters are often manufactured from protein constituents, amino acids. A way of raising the level of chemical good mood mediators is to increase intake of precursor amino acids, such as tryptophan for serotonin. This amino acid is found in spirulina, which is an alga, soyabeans, poultry liver, turkey, chicken, tofu, almonds.

• Eat fatty fish (sardines, mackerel, salmon) three times a week. It contains long-chain omega-3 fatty acids which have proven their efficacy against the symptoms of depression (*read the inset*).

• Sport has an effect on mental state by increasing the levels of form and good mood brain hormones.

My phytotherapeutic advice

St John's wort is an excellent plant antidepressant that has long been recognised. This plant has been the subject of a large number of clinical trials (more than 65 scientific papers). All of them prove its efficacy in cases of slight or moderate

Dietary supplements

Omega-3: for people who do not like fish, fish oil capsules are available at pharmacies and parapharmacies.

Vitamin B9: several studies have demonstrated a shortage of vitamin B9 in depressed people. In case of mood disorders, take a course of folic acid (400 mg to 1 mg per day).

depression and especially its perfect tolerance. St John's wort is also indicated in the context of withdrawal of antidepressants.

Pitfalls to avoid

Nicotine has an analgesic and antidepressant effect. It regulates mood and decreases anxiety by stimulating dopamine and serotonin secretion. If your mood barometer is not set on fine and sunny, it is certainly not the time to stop smoking (it would accentuate the depressed feeling), but be careful not to smoke more.

The psych war

Newspapers and magazines often publish articles on the psych war. This profession is indeed poorly defined. Between psychiatrists, psychoanalysts, psychologists and other psychotherapists, patients wanting to find a solution to their health or personality problems are lost and are never quite sure whether the professional they are consulting is a doctor or not.

To us, the matter is more simple. We believe that people who consult psychs very often have omega-3 fatty acid, vitamin and potassium deficiencies. And practising psychotherapy without taking the patients' dietary status into account, and their possible deficiencies, is simply not medicine.

Omega-3 fatty acids; good for morale

These fatty acids, known for their beneficial effects on the cardiovascular system, may also improve the symptoms of depression.

More than 60% of the weight of the brain consists of fats and more than 70% of these fats are omega-3 fatty acids. The latter would seem to have a degree of responsibility for the onset of depression. Indeed, depressives show a serious shortage of omega-3 fatty acids, particularly the very long-chain EPA and DHA[54]. This imbalance makes them very susceptible. In the nerve cells, it leads to a decrease in the receptors responsible for receiving the chemical good mood messenger, serotonin. Deprived of serotonin, the body sinks more readily into depression[55] When EPA and DHA supplements (in addition to their treatment) are given to people under chronic stress or depressives, a clear improvement in their symptoms is noted in most cases[56]. Very often, amxiety, sleep and libido are also improved[57]. EPA (1 g/day) seems, in mood disorders, to be the most active principle. However, most of these studies were conducted while the patients continued to take their medication. It is not clearly known what happens when omega-3 fatty acids are used on their own.

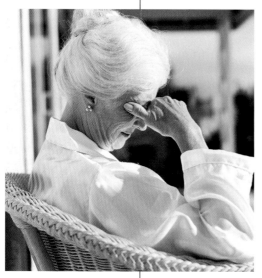

Health target
Fatigue

Less salt, more potassium: why?

To enable all our cells to eliminate the sodium that they contain, recover their normal size and re-start their metabolism. In this way, the cells will work better, they will again take in calories and this will restore energy.

My dietary advice

The health regimen suggested in this book is an excellent starting point.

• Generally speaking, eat just enough to satisfy your hunger; leave the table before starting to feel satiated. Having a light diet every day, allowing yourself an extra from time to time, is the right attitude.

• Eat at least five fresh plant products per day, either as vegetables or as fruit. Vegetables must be the basis of the diet, it is the best way of taking advantage of their hundreds of constituents and notably the potassium that they contain.

• Above all, have a varied diet, don't eat the same thing all the time.

• Inactivity makes you tired! Regular physical activity is the best assurance of good form.

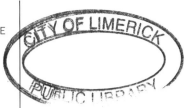

My phytotherapeutic advice

Plants high in polyphenols, effective against excess weight, are also effective against fatigue. I would recommend two: maté and green tea extract.

Maté is a plant that has not been used for long in Europe but is very well known in South America, where it is regularly drunk (like coffee here). Medicinal use of maté to combat mental and physical fatigue is recognised. The theophylline and caffeine present in the leaves stimulate the cardiac muscle and the central nervous system, relax the smooth muscles and have a good effect on peripheral blood circulation.

Tea is also a well-known central nervous system stimulant. It contains caffeine and polyphenols in very large quantities. It promotes both mental and muscular effort.

Pitfalls to avoid

Ladies, watch your iron. One-quarter of women between the age of puberty and the menopause have an iron shortage, a deficiency which gives rise to persistent fatigue if it is not corrected. To feel your energy returning, eat liver and red meat.

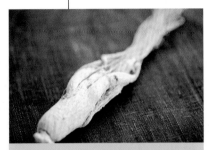

A remedy for fatigue: ginseng

Ginseng is a natural stimulant that does not have the harmful effects of excitants such as caffeine or amphetamines. It has toning and harmonising action. It stimulates mental and physical energy. It is a plant to use when you feel tired because you are working too hard, when you are always rushing to catch up, or when morale gets low. Ginseng makes it possible to keep your energy intact under lifestyle conditions that generate fatigue. It is an excellent restorative during convalescence after an operation or a debilitating viral infection. This is one of the indications most widely-recognised in the scientific community. Its action is greater when it is combined with vitamins.

Menopause

Less salt, more potassium: why?

At the menopause, women lose the protective effect that estrogens had exerted until then on the heart, vessels and blood lipids. In fact, at the age of 50, women generally see their bad cholesterol level increase, their blood pressure rise and, very often, weight piles on. By reducing salt in the diet and increasing the potassium intake, the cholesterol level, blood pressure and weight are more easily controlled. Moreover, microcirculation is improved, which limits hot flushes and night sweats.

Phytoestrogens: natural molecules that are beneficial during the menopause

Plants naturally produce substances which, once ingested, fix on the same receptors as female hormones. They are known as phytoestrogens, although their estrogenic activity is very slight (one-thousandth of that of estradiol). In the 1950s, two of these substances were isolated: genistein and daidzein, which are isoflavones. Soya, for example, is exceptionally high in genistein and daidzein. Soya isoflavones provide many benefits for the health and wellbeing of menopausal women. These benefits have been identified by epidemiological studies; some have since been confirmed by clinical trials. These isoflavones are very successfully used in the menopause in all the countries of the world.

My dietary advice

At the menopause, women will derive great benefit from foods high in phytoestrogens (*read the inset*). Where can these substances be found?

They are divided into three big families:

- **isoflavones:** mainly present in legumes, notably soyabeans, but also in chick peas, French beans, tea, etc.
- **lignans:** in whole cereal grain, oilseeds (flax, olives, sunflower), in flageolets, lentils, cherries, apples, pears, grapefruit, garlic, etc.

- **coumestans**, with a structure close to that of isoflavones, are found in lucerne (alfalfa) and particularly in soya shoots

• **Hot flushes:** several clinical trials [58, 59] have clearly shown the efficacy of soya isoflavones against hot flushes. A daily intake of 40 to 80 mg makes it possible to reduce their incidence and their severity.

• **Prevention of cardiovascular disease:** soya isoflavones significantly reduce "bad" cholesterol (LDL) and triglycerides, and increase "good" cholesterol (HDL).

• **revention of cancer of the breast,** the ovaries, the endometrium: the incidence of these cancers is 5 to 20 times lower in populations which have a high-phytoestrogen diet. Soya intake is associated with a reduced risk of breast cancer.[60]

• **Prevention of osteoporosis:** some studies suggest that isoflavones slow bone loss.

Pitfalls to avoid

Beware of alcoholic drinks and spices; they dilate the vessels and are liable to aggravate hot flushes

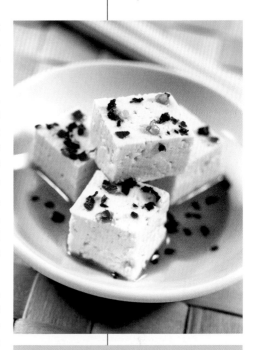

How to raise your isoflavone level?

In Europe, it is estimated that the average isoflavone intake is 1 mg/day, whereas it is 20 to 100 mg/day in Asia. Soya is incontestably the major source. As a guide, there are 20 mg of isoflavones in a glass of soya milk or in 65 g of tofu. Finally, dietary supplements based on high-isoflavone soya extracts (**Phytosoya**®)®) are available at pharmacies and parapharmacies. The recognised active dose of soya isoflavone is between 70 and 80 mg per day.

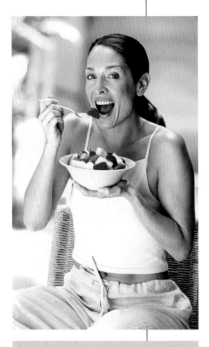

Soya isoflavones

Several studies have shown that by taking an isoflavone supplement, it is possible to slow bone mass loss in postmenopausal women. A recently-published study seems to confirm this: 177 women aged between 49 and 65 were divided into two groups. The first took 43 mg a day of isoflavones for one year, the second a placebo. At the end of the study, the women who had taken the isoflavones saw their bone mineral density in the lumbar vertebrae increase[61].

Osteoporosis

Less salt, more potassium: why?

By reducing dietary salt and increasing potassium intake, the body's acid-base equilibrium is restored, urinary elimination of calcium is reduced and bone resorption is slowed.

My dietary advice

To combat osteoporosis, the body must first of all be supplied with adequate quantities of calcium (1 g/day) but this is not enough. Calcium absorption, retention and fixation depend heavily on numerous parameters: the acid-base equilibrium, the presence of vitamin D and physical activity.

- Eat a lot of **fruit and vegetables**: they provide potassium and magnesium but also phytoestrogens and polyphenols, molecules known for their antioxidant properties; they can slow bone loss.

- Eat less meat. Animal proteins acidify the blood and oblige the body, in order to restore the acid-base equilibrium, to take calcium from its reserves, i.e. the bones.

- Watch your **vitamin D** levels. Small amounts of this vitamin are supplied by the diet (cod liver oil, fatty fish, egg yolk). The body obtains it above all from exposure to

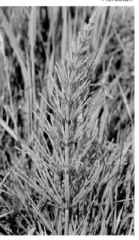

Horsetail

sunlight (the skin produces it from cholesterol due to the effect of ultraviolet rays).

• Keep active. Sedentary people lost more calcium than people who regularly pursue **physical activity**. Exercise plays an important part in bone remodelling. The resulting traction exerted by the muscles and the increase in muscle mass stimulate bone activity. All sports are good except perhaps for swimming since it does not make it possible to exert sufficient pressure on the bone.

My phytotherapeutic advice

Bamboo and **horsetail** are two plants that are very high in silica. Silica is a mineral that, on its own, makes it possible for the body to fix calcium, phosphorus and magnesium. It promotes absorption but also fixation in the bony tissues.

Pitfalls to avoid

While dairy products are indeed very high in calcium, they must not be abused. Cheeses are usually very salty. Milk in liquid form acidifies and therefore demineralises. Yoghurt is to be preferred. Fortunately, alongside milk products, there are many ways of obtaining calcium, for example by eating cruciferous vegetables (100 g of Chinese cabbage provides more calcium than a glass of milk).

Sources of calcium in a health diet (mg/100g)

Natural yoghurt	140-170
Fresh sardines	290
Almonds	250
Soya beans (mung beans)	255
Fresh parsley	200
Prawns	200
Cress	160
Walnuts and hazelnuts	175
Dried figs	160
Green olives	100
Cooked spinach	256
Endive	100
Cooked broccoli	100
Egg yolk	140
Cooked haricot beans	60
Cooked red kidney beans	112

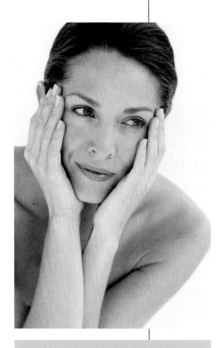

From time to time, take a course of antioxidants

To slow the rate of ageing and reduce the risk of age-associated illnesses, an antioxidant complex containing vitamins and minerals can be used. Select a supplement that provides beta-carotene, vitamin E, vitamin C, selenium and zinc.

Ageing

Less salt, more potassium: why?

Na/K pumps are omnipresent in the body. According to the organ concerned, there may be between 800,000 and 3 million pumps per cell. Restoring adequate sodium and potassium supplies means that these pumps will have better working conditions. They will be more efficient and will spare the cells from premature ageing.

My dietary advice

• Vary the pleasure by choosing the foods that are highest in protective components and lowest in components that accelerate ageing. The health regimen that we suggest conforms entirely to this principle.

Protective components: monounsaturated omega-3 fatty acids, sugars with a low glycemic index, carotenoids, vitamin C, vitamin E, polyphenols, potassium, calcium, magnesium, zinc, selenium, silicon.

Components that accelerate ageing: excessive saturated fats, sugars with a high glycemic index, sodium, chlorine, excessive iron and copper.

• Prepare food so as to retain all the protective components and not to produce any toxic components that accelerate ageing. In general, avoid very high temperature cooking (grilling, frying) and do not heat oils to smoking point.

• Do not force yourself to finish what is on your plate, and even less what is in the dish.

• With age, bone density and strength decrease progressively, as do the size and strength of the muscles. Regular, varied physical activity can help to overcome this physical decline. Moreover, it has a more general effect on the body's rate of ageing.

• As for the brain, it only wears out if you don't use it. The need for daily brain exercise must be emphasized.

Our enemies, free radicals

Our bodies need energy to function properly. The cell converts the nutrients provided by the diet into energy and water. This conversion generates about 2% of oxygen molecules with an electron missing, which makes them very reactive. These molecules, called free radicals, cause great damage in the cell and are at the root of cell ageing. Free radicals are also generated by external attack. A poor diet, stress, medication, the sun's rays, pollution, smoking, alcohol, microbial attacks, etc., accelerate free radical production in the body.

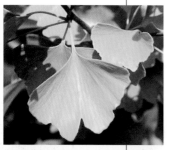

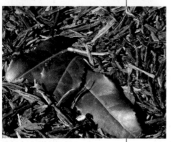

Ginkgo biloba and tea

My phytotherapeutic advice

Plants are full to bursting with antioxidant compounds that protect the body from the harmful effects of free radicals (*see inset on p. 97*): flavonoids. Many plants will thus act against ageing.

Ginkgo biloba increases blood circulation in the brain and, through its antioxidant properties, protects it against ageing. Ginkgo improves the memory but also the sight, by irrigating the retinas, and it prevents auditory senescence.

All veinotonic plants provide large quantities of flavonoids: **red vine**, **butcher's broom**, **sweet clover**, **hamamelis**, **cypress**, **horse chestnut**. This also applies to **olive leaves**, **lesser periwinkle** and **tea** extract.

Pitfalls to avoid

• Avoid toxins: tobacco, alcohol, pollution and heavy metals such as mercury and lead, that accelerate ageing.
• Avoid sudden, intensive or prolonged exposure to sunlight.

Finally, what to do about our skin?

After our long journey through our cells, that give us life and health, their high-potassium composition and their ceaseless struggles to defend themselves against sodium invasion, the difficult balancing act needed to stay hydrated, neither too turgescent nor too desiccated, what about our skin, that organ that envelops our body, that protects us from cold, wind, rain and sun. Yes, what about our skin?

Well! Our skin, too, has to have enough potassium for the cells of the dermis, which are constantly renewed, to operate the Na/K pump that ensures their equilibrium.

This is why it is useful for our diet to contain potassium and Na/K pump activators (saponins, flavonoids), antioxidants, vitamins and minerals. Locally, it is sensible to use cosmetics high in plant extracts, potassium, saponins, omega-3 fatty acids, which will enable all the cells in our skin to renew themselves, to stay young, to have good blood circulation (no blotchiness), to remain supple and elastic, keep wrinkles away for as long as possible.

One range of cosmetics has all the elements we have just mentioned, plant extracts, saponins, flavonoids high in potassium and antioxidants. That is the **Plant**

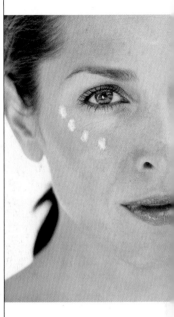

Dead Sea salts

On the shores of the Dead Sea, in Israel, spas have been created where visitors bathe in water saturated with Dead Sea salts. Courses of treatment improve the state of the skin and cure psoriasis. In Europe and America, sachets of dehydrated Dead Sea salts are available to take the cure in your own bathroom. You need to know that the waters of the Dead Sea contain a very large amount of potassium salts and a little sodium.

It is therefore easy to understand that the waters of the Dead Sea are beneficial to skin health. But the same activity can be obtained from cosmetics high in potassium and antioxidants (olive tree leaf, tea and sea buckthorn extract).

HOW
DID WE GET TO THIS POINT?

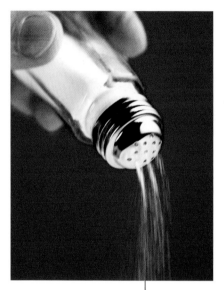

There has been a long, slow change in our dietary habits, combined with widespread failure to understand our body's mineral composition.

1. We were very slow to understand the distinctive composition of our high-potassium, low-sodium cells. It was Professors Albert Lehninger, Melvin J. Fregly and a few others who realised how much our body depended on potassium for the life of its cells. It is they who came up with the notion, to explain this high potassium content, that our cells had taken on the composition of an early Precambrian sea, at the time when the first living cells came into being. Then, over thousands and thousands of years, the sea's formula changed, its sodium content increased, but our cells did not alter theirs.

2. We did not take account of Paleolithic man's diet, either. Our ancestors had a very different diet from our own, and notably, they took in a lot of potassium and little sodium.

3. We had no concept of what, on page 12, I have called The Fight for Life. How do fish and marine mammals, whose blood contains 9 g of salt per litre whereas they ceaselessly swallow sea water, which contains 30 to 38 g of salt per litre, manage to regulate their blood composition?

In the light of our cells' special composition, we did not understand the battle that they wage, ceaselessly irrigated as they are by high-sodium, low-potassium blood, whereas they contain very little sodium and 28 times more potassium than the blood.

4. We therefore failed to realise that the fact of ceaselessly supplying our body with a lot of sodium and little potassium was exhausting it. In this fight for life, our cells have great difficulty in retaining their very special composition and this is what explains all those metabolic illnesses which are developing and which endanger our health and the very existence of humanity.

We talk endlessly about the danger of AIDS to the world but nobody has ever mentioned this far greater danger which is putting part of humanity in peril.

What has made everything worse is that man has developed a taste for salt, little by little, and salt is found in all foods, even sweet cakes, because salt enhances flavour. Then to please their customers and because salt improves the texture of all foods, the food industry put a lot of salt in all prepared foods. Cooks have also got into this habit and all dishes served in restaurants have had salt added when they reach your table. Salt is everywhere.

We wanted to expose this state of affairs and after two years of study and compiling a considerable bibliography, we were able to show, supported by clinical trials, that excess salt (and a lack of potassium) was at the root of all the XXL syndrome illnesses.

So what do we do now?

The public, the medical profession and government authorities had to be informed of the dangers of salt (and a lack of potassium). That is the purpose of this book. All consumers must now be informed about what they are eating. The amount of added salt must be stated on all foods.
Do you know that bread is highly salted?
How much salt there is in bacon? In all frozen meals or canned foods?

We do not think foods should be labelled like cigarettes, **SALT KILLS** but we have to know the amount of salt they contain.

Graham MacGregor, in his book **Salt, Diet and Health** gives an example of the label on a packet of breakfast cereal. This cereal contains 230 mg of sodium per 21 g of cereal. 230 mg of sodium is 575 mg of salt (NaCl) which means that this cereal contains as much salt as seawater does.

Which of us has not inadvertently swallowed a mouthful of sea water while swimming? It's not pleasant, yet any food that contains 3% salt is as salt as the sea.

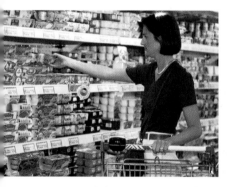

WHO Recommendations

We close with a word about the global health plan that has just been published by the WHO, the World Health Organisation (April 2004).

After months of negotiations, in April 2004 the 192 WHO nations approved a global plan to help millions of people to avoid obesity and many other chronic illnesses (according to us, they are the illnesses of the XXL syndrome) by adopting certain dietary rules: the WHO recommends limiting intake of saturated fats, trans fatty acids (contained in margarine), sugar and salt in prepared foods. The WHO asks all food companies to adopt responsible marketing strategies and to adhere to clear labelling for the foods that they manufacture in order to help the consumer to be better informed and to decide to buy healthy foods.

The WHO decisions have our 100% approval and we hope that the authorities in all the countries (192 nations) will apply this Directive as soon as possible.

The WHO has not said that in addition, potassium should be taken because we are all short of it. All these decisions are important to the health of future generations.

CONCLUSION

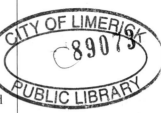

As we come to the end of this book, we want to record a disquieting fact:

All the scientific facts related in this book were found in books on biochemistry, physiology and in scientific papers compiled by eminent professors – the Na/K pump was discovered more than 50 years ago by eminent scientists, some of whom were awarded the Nobel Prize for their remarkable discoveries.

And despite all these discoveries, which have remained the secret garden of a few scientific circles, the medical profession, health professionals and the pharmaceutical industry have remained outside these great discoveries. This applies to the food industry, too, which has continued and still continues putting insane amounts of salt in food without giving a thought to the dramatic consequences that this may have for public health.

We wanted to disclose these discoveries and make them widely known so that future generations may have the benefit of what is best for their health.

We are not trying for the Novel Prize, even though we might wonder whether doing good to humanity does not merit the Nobel Prize?

INDEX

BIBLIOGRAPHY

1. JI Mann and AS Truswell (ed.) *Essentials of Human Nutrition*, Oxford University Press, Oxford, 2002, p 111.

2. Anthony D. C. Macknight and Alexander Leaf: *Regulation of cellular volume*. Physiological reviews,1977; vol 57, (3) : 510-573.

3. Greger R., Windhorst U. : *Cell volume In Comprehensive human physiology from cellular mechanisms to integration*, Springer-Verlag, Berlin, 1996, p 1360-136.

4. Naismith DJ : *The effect of low-dose potassium supplementation on blood pressure in apparently healthy volunteers*. Br J Nutr 2003 Jul;90(1):53-60.

5. Green DM : *Serum potassium level and dietary potassium intake as risk factors for stroke*. Neurology 2002 Aug 13;59:314-20.

6. Langfield MRW : *Salt and left ventricular hypertrophy: what are the links ?* J Human Hypertens 1995;9:909-916.

7. Cohn JN : *New guidelines for potassium replacement in clinical practice. A contemporary review by the National Council on Potassium in Clinical Practice*. Arch Intern Med 2000;160 : 2429-36.

8. Leier CV : *Clinical relevance and management of the major electrolyte abnormalities in congestive heart failure : hyponatremia, hypokaliema and hypomagnesia*. Am Heart J 1994;128 : 564-574.

9. Tobian L : *Athero-sclerotic cholesterol ester deposition is markedly reduced with a high-potassium diet*. Journal of Hypertension. Suppl, 1989;7(6):S244-245.

Ishimitsu T : *High potassium diets reduce macrophage adherence to the vascular wall in stroke-prone spontaneously hypertensive rats*. J Vasc Res. 195 Nov-Dec;32(6):406-12

Ma G : *Inverse relationship between potassium intake and coronary artery disease in the cholesterol-fed rabbit*. Am J Hypertens. 199 Aug;12(8Pt 1):821-5

Young DB : *Vascular protective effects os potassium*. Senim Nephrol. 199 Sept;19(5):477-86

Tobian L : *High K diets markedly reduce atherosclerotic cholesterol ester deposition in aortas of rats with hypercholesterolemia and hypertension*. Am J Hypertens. 1990 Feb;3(2):133-5

10. White RE : *Estrogen relaxes coronary arteries by opening BKCa channels through a cGMP-dependent mechanism.* Circ Res, 1995 ; 77:936-942.

11. Rusko J : *17-_-Estradiol stimulation of endothelial K^+ channels.* Biochemical and Biophysical research communication. 1995 vol 214;n°2 :367-372.

12. Darkow DJ : *Estrogen relaxation of coronary artery smooth muscle in mediated by Nitric Oxyde and cGMP.* Am J. Physiol, 1997; 272 (Heart circ Physiol 41) H 2765-H2773.

13. Wellman GC : *Gender differences in coronary artery diameter involve Estrogen, Nitric Oxide and $Ca\_^+$ dependent K^+ channels.* Circ Res, 1996;79 :1024-1030.

14. De Luise M. : *Reduced activity of red-cell sodium-potassium pump in human obesity.* The New England Journal of Medicine, 1980;303 : 1017-1022.

15. Rowe JW : *Effect of experimental potassium deficiency on glucose and insulin metabolism.* Metabolism 1980;29 : 498-502.

16. Helderman JH : *Prevention of the glucose intolerance of thiazide diuretics by maintenance of the body potassium.* Diabetes 1983;32 : 106-111.

17. Donovan DS : *Effect of sodium intake on insulin sensitivity.* Am J Physiol 1993;264: E730-E734.

18. Ogihara T : *Contribution of salt intake to insulin resistance associated with hypertension.* Life Sciences 2003;509-523.

19. Ogihara T : *High salt diet enhances insulin signalling and induces insulin resistance in Dahl salt-sensitive rats.* Hypertension 2002;40:83-89.

20. Ogihara T : *Insulin resistance with enhanced insulin signalling in high salt diet fed rats.* Diabetes 2001;50 : 573-583.

21. El-Mallakh RS : *The Na,K-ATPase hypothesis for bipolar disorder : implication for normal development.* J Child Adolescent Psychopharmacol, 1993;3 : 37-52.

22. Pontzer NJ : *Receptors, phosphoinositol hydrolisis and plasticity of nerve cells.* Prog Brain Res 1990;86 : 221-225.

23. Webb WL : *Electrolyte and fluid imbalance : neuropsychatric manifestations.* Psychosomatics, 1981;22(3):229-233.

24. Burney P : *A diet rich in sodium may potentiate asthma. Epidemiologic evidence for a new hypothesis.* Chest. 1987;91(Suppl.):143S-148S.

25. Lindahl O : *Vegan regimen with reduced medication in the treatment of bronchial asthma.* Journal of asthma, 1985;22:45-55.

26. Joosens JV : *Dietary salt, nitrate and stomach cancer mortality in 24 countries. European cancer Prevention (ECP) and the INTERSALT Cooperative Research group.* Int J Epidemiol 1996;25: 494-504.

27. Terry P : *Protective effect of fruits and vegetables on stomach cancer in a cohort of Swedish twins.* International Journal of Cancer, 1998;76:35-37.

28. Sriamporn S : *Gastric cancer : the roles of diet, alcohol drinking, smoking and Helicobacter pylori in Northeastern Thailand.* Asian Pac J cancer Prev 2002;3(4):345-352.

29. Villanueva CM : *Meta-analysis of studies on individual consumption of chlorinated drinking water and bladder cancer.* J Epidemiol Community Health 2003;57(3):166-173.

30. Ruffié Jacques : *Naissance de la médecine prédictive.* Odile Jacob, 1993.

31. Burnet RB : *Chronic fatigue syndrome: is total body potassium important ?* Med J Aust. 1996;164(6):384.

32. Fraser S : *Fatigue depresses maximal in vitro skeletal muscle Na^+-$K+$-ATPase activity in untrained and trained individuals.* J Appl Physiol 2002;93: 1650-1659.

33. Barzel US : *The skeleton as an ion exchange system : implications for the role of acid-base imbalance in the genesis of osteoporosis.* J Bone Miner Res 1995;10 : 1431-1436.

34. Eaton BS : *An evolutionary perspective enhances understanding of human nutritional requirements.* J Nutr 1996;126 : 1732-1740.

35. New SA : *Dietary influences on bone mass and bone metabolism : further evidence of a positive link between fruit and vegetable consumption and bone health ?* Am J Clin Nutr 2000;71 : 142-151.

36. Lin PH : *The DASH diet and sodium reduction improve markers of bone turnover and calcium metabolism in adults.* J Nutr 2003;133(10) : 3130-6.

37. Sebastian A : *Improved mineral balance and skeletal metabolism in postmenopausal women treated with potassium bicarbonate.* The New England Journal of Medicine 1994;330 : 1776-1781.

38. Devine A : *A longitudinal study of the effect of sodium and calcium intakes on regional bone density in postmenopausal women.* Am J Clin Nutr 1995;62: 740-745.

39. Matkovik V : *Urinary calcium, sodium and bone mass of young females.* Am J Clin Nutr 1995; 62:417-25.

40. Poehlman ET : *Regulation of energy expenditure in aging humans.* Geriatr Biosci 1993;41 : 552-559.

41. Harik SI : *Ouabain binding in the human brain. Effects of Alzheimer's disease and aging.* Arch Neurol 1989;46(9):951-954.

42. Yi Li : *The discovery of novel openers of Ca$^+$-dependent large-conductance potassium channels : pharmacophore search and physiological evaluation of flavonoids,* Bioorganic & Med Chemistry Letters, Elsevier Science Ltd, Great Britain, 1997,7(7) : 759-762.

43. Eaton SB : *Paleolithic nutrition revisited : A twelve-year retrospective on its nature and implications.* Eur J Clin Nutr 1997;51 : 207-216.

44. Elliott P : *The INTERSALT study : results for 24 hour sodium and potassium, by age and sex. INTERSALT Co-operative Research Group.* J Hum Hypertens 1989;3(5) : 323-330.

45. Jansson B : *Dietary, total body and intracellular potassium-to-sodium ratios and their influence on cancer.* cancer Detect Prev 1990;14(5) : 563-565.

46. Food and Nutrition Board, Institute of Medicine. Potassium. *Dietary Reference Intakes for Water, Potassium, Sodium, Chloride, and Sulfate.* National Academies Press, Washington DC, 2004 :173-246.

47. Hunt JF : *Endogenous airway acidification. Implications for asthma pathophysiology.* Am J Respir Crit Care Med, 2000;61 : 694-699.

48. Vats V : *Evaluation of anti-hyperglycemic and hypoglycemic effect of Trigonella foenum-graecum Linn, Ocimum sanctum Linn and Pterocarpus marsupium Linn in normal and alloxanized diabetic rats.* J of Ethno-Pharm, 2002;79:95-100.

49. Agrawal P : *Randomized placebo-controlled, single blind trial of holy basil leaves in patients with noninsulin-dependent diabetes mellitus.* Inter Journ of Clini Pharma and Therap 1996;Vol. 34, N°9 : 406-409

50. Chattopadhyay RR : *Hypoglycemic effect of Ocimum sanctum leaf extract in normal and streptozotocin diabetic rats.* Indian Jour of Exp Biology,1993;Vol.31 : 891-893

51. Rai V : *Effect of Tulsi (Ocimum sanctum) leaf powder supplementation on blood sugar levels, serum lipids and tissue lipids in diabetic rats.* Plant Foods for Human Nutrition, 1997;50 : 9-16

52. Anghsula Sarkar : *Changes in the blood lipid profile after administration of ocimum sanctum (tulsi) leaves in the normal albino rabbits*, Indian J Physiol Pharmacol 1994;38(4) : 311-312.

53. Bennani-Kabchi N : *Therapeutic effect of Olea europea var. oleaster leaves on carbohydrate and lipid metabolism in obese and prediabetic sand rats (Psammomys obesus).* Ann Pharm Fr, 2000;58(4) : 271-277.

54. Peet M : *Depletion of omega-3 fatty acid levels in red blood cell membranes of depressive patients.* Biol Psychiatry, 1998;43 : 315-319.

55. Simopoulos AP : *Omega-3 fatty acids in inflammation and autoimmune diseases.* J Am Coll Nutr 2002;21(6) : 495-505.

56. Locke CA : *Omega-3 fatty acids in major depression.* World Rev Nutr Diet. 2001;89:173-185.

57. Peet M : A *dose-ranging study of the effects of ethyl-eicosapentaenoate in patients with ongoing depression despite apparently adequate treatment with standard drugs.* Arch Gen Psychiatry. 2002, 59(10) : 913-919.

58. Albertazzi P : *The effect of dietary soy supplementation on hot flushes.* Obstet Gynecol 1998;91 : 6-11.

59. Scambia G. : *Clinical effects of a standardized soy extract in postmenopausal women : a pilot study.* Menopause 2000;7 : 105-111.

60. Yamamoto S : *Soy, isoflavones and breast cancer risk in Japan.* Journal of the National Cancer Institute 2003;95(12) : 906-913.

61. Atkinson C : *The effects of phytoestrogen isoflavones on bone density in women : a double-blind, randomised, placebo-controlled trial.* Am J Clin Nutr, 2004;79(2) : 326-333.

Books

Lehninger : *Principles of Biochemistry*. 3rd ed, Worth Publishers, N Y , 2000.

Andreoli T : *Physiology of membrane disorders*. 2nd ed, Plenum Medical Book Cie, N Y, 1986.

Devlin T : *Textbook of biochemistry*. 5th ed, Wiley & Sons, Inc, NY, 2002.

Alberts B : *Essential Cell Biology*, Garland Publishing Inc, New York & London, 1998.

Loddish Berk : *Molecular Cell Biology*. 5th ed, Freeman, England, 1986.

Boyton H, McCarty MF, Moore RD : *The salt solution*. Avery Publishing Group, New York, 2001.

Reaven G : Syndrome X : *overcoming the silent killer that can give you a heart attack*. Simon & Schuster, New York, 2000.

MacGregor GA, Wardener HE : *Salt, Diet and Health*, Cambridge University Press, Cambridge, 1998.

In our collection Alpen Éditions:

-The Omega-3 Answer

-Living with a Hyperactive Child

-All About the Prostate

-The French Paradox

-The XXL Syndrome

with Michel Montignac:

-Eat Yourself Slim

-The Montignac Diet Cookbook

-The French GI Diet

-Glycemic Index Diet

www.alpen.mc